Clothed in W[...]

D0181664

C/BC

CLOTHED
IN
WHITE

"For to me to live is Christ, and to die is gain."

RAY G. REGISTER, JR.

BROADMAN PRESS
NASHVILLE, TENNESSEE

© Copyright 1991 ● Broadman Press

4250-97
ISBN: 0-8054-5097-1
Dewey Decimal Classification: 266.092
Subject Heading: PATE, MAVIS // MISSIONS, MEDICAL //
MISSIONS - GAZA // MISSIONS - ORIENT
Library of Congress Card Catalog Number: 90-19870
Printed in the United States of America

Unless otherwise stated, Scripture quotations are from the *Revised Standard Version of the Bible*, copyrighted 1946, 1952, © 1971, 1973.
Scripture quotations marked KJV are from the *King James Version of the Bible*.

Library of Congress Cataloging-in-Publication Data

Register, Ray G.
  Clothed in white / Ray G. Register.
  p. cm.
  Includes bibliographical references and index.
  ISBN: 0-8054-5097-1 :
  1. Pate, Mavis Orisca, d. 1972. 2. Operating room nurses-
-Louisiana--Biography. 3. Missionaries, Medical--Developing
countries--Biography. 4. Hope (Hospital ship) I. Title.
  RD32.3.R44 1991
  610.73'092--dc20
  [B]

                                        90-19870
                                            CIP

*I dedicate this to missionary nurses
the world over who,
like Mavis did,
give of themselves unselfishly
for the healing and saving of others.*

Contents

Preface

God's Spirit moved powerfully throughout the churches in Israel, the West Bank, and Gaza during the early 1970s. Many national Christians and their missionary colleagues were caught up in the life-changing events during those exciting days. The tragic death of missionary nurse, Mavis O. Pate, in Gaza in 1972 caused us who witnessed these events to reflect on the cost of living for Christ and even the possibility of dying for Him. I have long felt that the life and impact of Mavis Pate—and the spiritual aftermath of her sacrifice—should be recorded. The Holy Spirit has constrained me to present Mavis's story.

In the Spring of 1979, I found myself in Ringgold, Louisiana, as a speaker in a World Missions Conference. I discovered that Mavis had grown up on a nearby farm. Her mother, Mattie Oden, showed me Mavis's letters and encouraged me to write her biography. I had the privilege of meeting Mavis's step-sister, Genie Norman, in Minden, Louisiana. They sent me a suitcase full of Mavis's personal correspondence via a tour group sponsored by Jack Taylor, well-known author-speaker. A thief stole the suitcase from a car in Tiberias and threw it into the Sea of Galilee, where the police retrieved it. The following morning I found the letters drying on the floor of the police station, fortunately in readable condition!

Years passed as mission duties kept me from giving more than limited time to the study of Mavis's correspondence. In June 1982, after attending the Southern Baptist Convention in New Orleans, I again visited Mattie Oden in Ringgold and met Gwen Lewis, Mavis's sister, in Shreveport, Louisiana. They shared personal memories of

Mavis, allowed me to read her life history written for the Foreign Mission Board, and introduced me to her friends.

Mavis wrote prolifically. She had a flair for absorbing the circumstances surroundings around her, and she wrote regular "round-robin" letters to her family. I have shared excerpts from these letters so you can have a personal part in her observations and adventures. I married a nurse and served in the U.S. Navy. So, I identified with her adventures on the *S.S. Hope*. Perhaps this, and the fact that I grew up in the country, caused me to be captivated by her letters and life. Above all, I attempt to present Mavis as I believe she would wish—*as a person on a pilgrimage to find a closeness and oneness with God in the service of mankind.* Her pilgrimage serves as the theme of this book.

I am deeply indebted to Mattie Oden, now deceased; Gwen Lewis, Genie Norman, their daughters, and friends who graciously granted me interviews. The former staff of the Gaza Baptist Hospital, especially Dr. Merrill Moore, Rev. Jarrell, Shirley Peach, Ava Nell McWhorter (R.N.), Lenore Mullican (R.N.), her husband Ken, and many others gave me interviews or wrote their impressions. Dr. Charles Beckett of the Bangladesh Baptist Mission and the staff of the Foreign Mission Board of the Southern Baptist Convention were especially helpful. Many helped me by proofreading and offering constructive comments, especially missionaries Ruth Rexrode Anderson and Elizabeth Smith. I am most grateful to my wife Rose Mary Register (R.N.) who offered me much "T.L.C." through these years of gathering information, writing, and rewriting.

1
Why Mavis?

Israeli Air Force jets practiced overhead, as usual, on Sunday, January 16, 1972, a reminder that war and violence are never far away in the Middle East. Galilee is normally peaceful, but the rumblings of the air ritual recalled memories of the 1967 June War. Evening approached. I wanted to relax with that dreamy feeling of "all's right with the world." Mist rolled over the hills surrounding the city as Rose Mary and I returned from evening services at the Nazareth Baptist Church. We expected rain to intensify the chill in our large stone house. As calm and peace settled around us I felt anticipation, but an unforgettably disturbing event shattered the tranquillity.

The phone rang. The voice on the other end reported: "Mavis has been shot. She's critical. Ed Nicholas has been wounded—but not severely. Pray for them." I hung up the phone and immediately prayed. Shortly the phone jangled again. The voice, more somber this time, announced, "Mavis is dead. There's nothing they could do. Funeral arrangements are being made. We'll be in touch."

My mind went momentarily berserk! *Mavis Pate dead? How could she be dead? I saw her just a few days ago at Baptist Village with that radiant smile on her face! How could this be?* "Dear Lord, Why Mavis?" Nothing allowed me to absorb the impact of this tragic news. But reality soon overcame my questioning.

While many friends and colleagues of Mavis slept fitfully, if at all, the Gaza Baptist Mission made late-night plans for her funeral. In the Middle East, burial is as hasty and almost as sudden as death. There is no embalming. Mavis left a specific request with her family when she was called overseas. If she died, she wanted to be buried in the land where she served.

The next morning, clear instructions arrived, "All friends of Mavis are to drive to the Israeli-Gaza border. There will be a special parking area. Under no circumstances are cars with Israeli license plates to be allowed into Gaza. A general curfew is in effect. Transportation will be provided from the border to the Gaza Baptist Hospital compound where the funeral is to be held."

Fear welled up in my heart. *Do we have to go to Gaza? They shot Mavis there only yesterday. What if there is an attack on a whole group of us?* My apprehensions were unfounded. As we approached the border, the military kept a high profile. The army sealed the border to all except those attending Mavis's funeral. After parking, we boarded the hospital bus. Missionary physiotherapist Jarrell Peach gave us directions. "We'll take an alternate route to the hospital compound from the one Mavis and Ed took yesterday. Return to the bus after the funeral, and they'll bring you back here." I admired Jarrell's composure. His command of a dreadfully tense situation inspired confidence.

The bus lumbered past the citrus orchards into the outskirts of Gaza Town. This time, my eyes neither noticed the dirt and the potholes in the road nor the greasy auto axles and motors spilling out of the auto repair garages. The staff, missionaries, and townspeople awaited our arrival before we gathered into the church on the compound. The sun peeked out from behind the clouds.

As we stood silently, the nursing students filed past, carrying wreaths decorated with ribbons bearing Mavis's name. We followed them into the church. An Israeli girl soldier walked ahead of me. An army officer mixed in with the Arab dignitaries from Gaza. *Strange,* I wondered, *How they hate each other, but now in the death of this Christian foreigner, they are drawn together! Is this what it takes to get Jew and Arab together?*

I sat down on the right side of the church. The satin-covered coffin smothered in flowers lay before the pulpit. An oversized picture of Mavis was placed on top. The full impact of the tragedy began to hit me.

Fighting back the tears, I listened as Roy McGlamery, hospital administrator, gave a short eulogy. Martha Murphey of Baptist Village in Israel sang "I Know That My Redeemer Liveth." Pastor Hanna Ibrahim from the Gaza Baptist Church spoke in Arabic. I had secretly admired his courage. Then Dr. Robert L. Lindsey, veteran Baptist representative from Jerusalem, stirred my heart as he read the words of Jesus in Luke 12:4-8: "Do not fear those who kill the body . . . even the hairs of your head are all numbered . . . everyone who acknowledges me before men, the Son of man will also acknowledge before the angels of God."

"Lord," I prayed, "Has Mavis made the ultimate sacrifice You may require of us all? Is this why You have allowed her to be taken so suddenly in the prime of life, by the hands of those whom she came to heal? Why Mavis, Lord? Why Mavis?"

The service closed as Rev. Jim Smith, Baptist representative from Ashkelon, committed Mavis to the Lord in prayer. Six male nurses lifted her coffin over their heads, bearing her away into the sunlight. Jarrell Peach requested that only the Gaza missionaries be present at the graveside. They felt like her family and wanted these last moments with her. That was my last memory of Mavis. But the question has haunted me through the years: "Why Mavis?"

2

Louisiana Beginnings

What made Brady Pate so popular with the girls? Was it his looks, his persistence, or his horse? "Brit" was a single-footing Louisiana country show horse. The older folks in Bienville and Red River parishes, Louisiana, still remember Brit and Brady courting the girls. "Brit's" famous gait became a regular sound on the road, every Sunday and Wednesday, to Mattie Bell Green's home. Mattie and Brady dated steadily for three years before the four-mile trip paid off. They married when he was twenty and she, eighteen.

As with many, hard times faced the young couple as they started life together. Mattie and Brady decided to borrow money from the Federal Land Bank of America. This enabled them to buy a small farm about five miles south of Ringgold, Louisiana. They started raising their family in a small clapboard house.

On October 20, 1923, their love rewarded them with the birth of a girl, Edna Gwendolyn. Two years later, Gwen's parents gave her an early Christmas present with the birth of a sister, Mavis Orisca, on December 23, 1925. Because of Mattie's ill health, Mavis weighed only 4 pounds and 2 ounces. Most of Mattie's energy went into rearing Mavis, leaving Brady to care for Gwen. Each girl acquired the dominant qualities of the parent who raised her.

Mavis inherited the Indian name "Orisca" from her paternal grandmother. Etta Orisca Cotter Pate, one-quarter Cherokee Indian from Oklahoma, was a tall, sensitive woman with high cheek bones and a reddish tinge to her hair. Not only her looks, but her spiritual life, influenced Mavis positively. Whenever life's turns perplexed, upset, or bewildered Etta, she had a way of stealing off to meditate and be alone with the Lord.

Brady's qualities of clean living and hard work were influences from his Irish father, Newton King Brady Pate. On their large farm, Brady grew up without learning to curse. His daughters remember the time he hit his head on the door, and all he could come up with was "Golly!" But if pushed too far, his Irish temper could flare up.

Brady had a favorite hunting dog who one day did not return home. He went out looking for him and found the dog had been shot in the back. He killed the poor animal to put it out of its misery. Then he went after the fellow who had done the shooting. When he confronted the man, Brady bit off half of his ear in the ensuing fist fight!

The Lord touched Brady about a year after Mavis was born. He accepted Christ during a revival and was baptized in Womack Creek, along with eight other converts. The family Bible nearly wore out from his reading it to the girls. He didn't smoke, curse, or even drink coffee in his lifetime.

How early can a girl know her life's calling? Mavis never found this a problem. At age three, she and her sister needed their tonsils removed. So, the family drove over to Shreveport in the Model-T Ford. On the way, Brady pulled up under the shade of an oak tree so Mattie could help the girls change into clean clothes. Then they headed for the hospital. Mavis fell so much in love with the nurses that she decided then and there to be a nurse! She never changed her mind.

In 1929 Brady Pate decided he needed to improve his education, selling his farm and settling Mattie and the girls near Ringgold. He headed for Chicago to study electrical engineering, a venture that almost cost his life. The bitter cold of Chicago degenerated his health, but he refused to go to the hospital. The doctor called Mattie and reported, "If Brady doesn't go back south he may die. He has severe cases of measles and pneumonia." Mavis's young age kept her from realizing the dire straits of her family and why they lived in a tenant house as sharecroppers. The Great Depression hit in 1929. As Mattie put it, "We just stayed one bubble above the water!" It challenged the Pates to keep body and soul together.

Growing Up—the Uninhibited Expression of Joy

Armadillos are strange-looking creatures to those unfamiliar with Louisiana, Mississippi, or the Southwest. They look like a cross between a dachshund and a turtle! You usually see them smashed on the highways because they're too dumb to get out of the way of cars! They dig up everything, rooting around with their long noses, looking for insects or roots, or whatever armadillos eat. When frightened, they roll up in their shells. Mavis was about five years old when Brady Pate caught an armadillo and tried to make it a pet. But it ended up smashed on the road like the rest of its friends!

Mavis was not one to crawl into her shell like a turtle. She grew up loving the farm with its horses and other animals. She went hunting and fishing with Brady. Mavis was always a bit tomboyish and also ambitious. With her sister Gwen's schoolbooks, she taught herself to read and write before she entered the first grade! From the time she entered elementary school early at the age of five years and nine months (in September 1930) she remained an "A" student. The Depression didn't make going to school easy. The Pates had no money to buy books and supplies, so Mavis and Gwen brought eggs from the farm and traded them for supplies at Woodard's store in Ringgold. It was a three-mile walk, one way, if you missed the school bus.

After Mattie nursed Brady back to health she became sick partly due to living in the dilapidated tenant house. Brady arose in the morning, cooked biscuits, and helped the girls get off to school before doing his chores. Every evening he read the big family Bible—with all the pictures—to his brood.

Most of their neighbors were blacks. It came as no surprise when those neighbors invited them to church at revival time. The girls were a bit apprehensive because they heard the blacks tended to shout when they "got happy" about their religion. When they arrived the Pates sat toward the back. To their surprise, the preacher called them down to the front as the honored guests for the evening.

When Mavis was in the second grade at Ringgold Grammar School the Lord began working on her conscience. She stole some chewing gum. The guilt was painful. She was also paddled for seat-jumping.

Mavis later wrote, "The resulting punishment curbed to a degree my uninhibited expression of joy in life."[1]

Farm life had its frustrations. Brady worked in timber during the winter. One day he came home to find the climbing cow missing. Yes, *a climbing cow!* She even climbed up into barns. The family always feared what that agile bovine might do to itself on one of its climbing escapades. In the bitter cold, Brady and the girls rode horses and searched far and wide all day. Finally they found the poor cow dead in a cotton house, her foot stuck in a hole between the boards.

Mavis always enjoyed reading more than doing farm work. She read every book she could find. Perhaps that was why she got into mischief when she had to do chores. One time, as they were stacking wood, she hit Gwen on the head with a piece of stovewood. Fortunately, it didn't knock her out! It seems that Mavis felt "put upon" because Gwen had an allergy and couldn't milk the cows.

Mavis found working cotton particularly tedious. Brady plowed and the women chopped cotton with the hoes. Mattie and Gwen worked their heads off and Mavis, back down the row, leaned on her hoe and looked up at the birds! Mattie thought, *She must be looking at the Lord. She stumbles over whatever is on the ground because she always looks up!* As she grew older Mavis became less placid. The neighbors still remember the sight of her riding on top of a load of cotton, driving a team of horses, on the way to the cotton gin.

Life on the farm rewarded Mavis and her family after they "laid by" the crops every year. Brady Pate loaded the family into the wagon and headed for Lake Bistineau (pronounced "Bristineau") for a week of camping and fishing. There Mavis ate her first frog legs. When it rained they turned the wagon bed over and crawled under it. During these family times Mavis excluded the outside world by curling up with a copy of *Swiss Family Robinson.*

The world could be violent during the Depression. The police ambushed "Bonnie and Clyde," the notorious bank robbers and murderers about five miles from Ringgold, just above the crossroads town of Jamestown in northwest Louisiana. They dragged their bullet-riddled car, with the warm bodies still inside, into a nearby school yard to prove to the youngsters that "crime does not pay."

The friendship of the Kings, a black family, meant a lot during those difficult years. They came over to the Pate's home and sang Gospel songs together in the evenings. Or the Kings would call out, "Why don't ya'll sing awhile tonight?" The Pate children played with blacks or they didn't play with anyone!

Mavis became increasingly aware of life's realities as she entered her teen years. What she experienced disturbed her. She found comfort in a most unusual place.

The Secret Place

The approach of the teenage years, of course, brought change into Mavis's life. When Grandma and Grandpa Pate died and the old Pate estate was divided among the children, Brady received his share of the land and managed to buy some additional land. The family moved to a new home three miles south of Ringgold.

New feelings stirred inside Mavis as she developed into a young lady and began to lose some of her tomboyish ways. In the sixth grade, she experienced her first case of "puppy love." She had a crush on the local banker's son. Little did she realize the anguish this would bring.

Years of Bible reading and going to church began to have an effect on her life. Mavis received Jesus as her personal Savior during a revival in the Spring of 1938 and was baptized in Womack Creek that May. She described her conversion as "more of a seeking of assurance of God's eternal love and eternal life than a conscious need of the forgiveness of sins." The Lord prepared her for what lay ahead.

Mavis traveled to another town to spend the night with some friends. She awoke in the night to the shock of the man of the house trying to fondle her body. She felt immediate revulsion. Pushing him away, she barricaded the door to her room. Needless to say, she didn't sleep the rest of the night! She feared to tell the man's wife or her father for fear of what he might do to the man. She thought, *Dad might kill him!* This event remained etched in her memory for years to come. She kept it to herself and didn't even share it with her mother or sister, not knowing at the time that this man subjected other girls to the same indignity.[2]

Seventh-grade graduation ushered in her teen years. The class prophecy predicted Mavis as an airline hostess. However, she knew better. "I'll be a nurse, no matter what my friends think," Mavis insisted.

At an eighth-grade school party she experienced her first kiss. She related, "I was infatuated with the boy, but I felt guilty about the kiss and found myself shy and withdrawn afterwards when around him. I did not understand myself, nor could I make myself act differently. I could not bring myself to discuss it with anyone. Needless to say, my first love was a very unhappy one!"[3]

Mavis coped with her teenage frustrations by immersing herself in school studies and sports activities. She played first base in softball. She also turned her thoughts toward the Lord. Her family began attending the Methodist church close to their home, but there were urges and impulses in her heart that she could not share with anyone else. *How can I handle this?* she pondered.

The big sycamore tree behind the barn offered the answer. The tree flecked off its bark in long brown patches. Even the animals felt secure under its shelter. Grandmother Orisca Pate had found solace when she became confused or perplexed by going out behind her house to pray. Mavis discovered her secret place. "I developed the habit about this time by choosing a secret place—a clump of trees in the meadow where I went to talk to God about my problems or just be alone with Him," she later related.[4]

And problems there were! By 1940 Mavis started dating, not seriously, or anything leading to marriage. She was not much for "spooning" as holding hands and kissing were called then. She and a neighbor boy began to date. Mavis became sensitive about her appearance. One day he came over unexpectedly and caught Mavis in her old work clothes milking a cow. She was mortified!

Mavis felt much more comfortable when her best friend Lormia Lee or "Lorie" was around. Lorie pitched on the girl's softball team. Mavis could catch any ball thrown to her. Lorie and Mavis double-dated, ran around together, and occasionally got into trouble.

War clouds hung over the world in the 1940s. Nazi Germany had conquered most of Europe. December 7, 1941, was "a day that will in infamy"—the Sunday when Japan made a surprise attack on the American fleet at Pearl Harbor. The United States was at war! "Bewilderment and deep distress were real emotions to me. I went to my place," related Mavis. War affected her future in an unexpected way.[5]

L. V. Noles, principal of Ringgold High School, remembers Mavis as a "quiet, non-aggressive kind of girl. She had a good attitude about life and a pleasant personality. She was not a loner. There was always a crowd around Mavis. We did not have a religious atmosphere in the school, but Mavis had within her the make-up that caused people in need to appeal to her."[6]

How Mavis acted after school hours was another story! Her Dad gave her a Model-A Ford four-door sedan to drive during the last two years of high school. By this time, he had recovered financially from the Depression. Mavis enjoyed taking their cook, Mrs. King, for a fling in the car. Despite all her social activities Mavis kept her school grades high. She was chosen to bring the valedictory address at the high-school graduation.

The Model-A Ford was her undoing! Despite all the freedom Brady and Mattie gave Mavis, one pastime they forbade—going to movies on Sunday. However, before graduation, she and Lorie felt that slipping out to the movies just one Sunday afternoon would do no harm. Returning from the movies, Lorie drove and Mavis sat in the back seat with a girl friend. Suddenly a drunk driver swerved in front of them! Crash!!! Lorie sideswiped the other car. Mavis received a blow on her head, leaving her face bruised. The tell-tale bruise kept Mavis from having her senior picture made.[7]

The war ushered prosperity into the Pate household, but it also fomented strife. Brady and Mattie worked separate shifts in an ordnance factory. Mavis noticed that they argued often. When this happened she left the room, buried herself in a book, or slipped away to the solitude of her "secret place." Mavis never understood why couples argued. *Why can't they settle their differences?* she thought. *There should be a simple solution to domestic problems.* One was not to be found in the Pate household.

Student Nursing—"Sturb"

Mavis's childhood dream came true when the North Louisiana School of Nursing in Shreveport waived the minimum age requirement for her. She entered nurses' training before her seventeenth birthday. The desire to keep up with her older sister, who also entered nursing, drove her. "If Gwen can do it, I can too!" was her motto.

Loretta Sturbenz, or "Sturb" as the students called her, supervised the operating room at the North Louisiana Sanitarium, later known as Doctor's Hospital. Sturb had the fortune to teach Mavis operating-room technique, and the misfortune, when off duty, to be the dormitory matron where the nurses lived. She knew Mavis as an excellent student with a positive spirit who asked questions and offered a few sound suggestions of her own.

But the girls, including Mavis, had a knack of slipping out at nights after curfew. Sturb wished they had oiled the squeaky fire escape because it always gave them away! She played along with them, knowing that they headed to the U.S.O. Nurses belonged to the Cadet Corps during World War II. The government subsidized their tuition and supplied their uniforms. The U.S.O. was only three blocks from the dormitory, and the girls "snuck" out to dance with the young servicemen. Sturb knew that seventeen-year-old girls were like "babes in the woods." Many a father told Sturb, "I feel my girl is safe with you." She spent many an anxious night waiting to hear the squeak of the fire escape as the girls tiptoed into the dorm![8]

While the added freedom was exhilarating to Mavis, it devastated her spiritual life. She later reflected, "My Christian life was almost non-existent during the next several years. I learned to dance from the girls in the dormitory and attended U.S.O. parties with the group. My knowledge of the Bible and Christian discipleship was very meager, and I felt no guilt in participating in these activities."[9]

During the U.S.O. escapades, Mavis struck up a friendship with one of the young servicemen there. Mavis thought he was nice, sincere, and considerate, but the relationship never developed. "When he was sent overseas several months later, I felt a warm concern for him but not the deep, abiding love that I felt would lead to marriage. We made no promises other than that we would see how things worked out when he returned."[10]

In 1943, Brady Pate made the last payment on his debts from the Depression, including the hospital bills. Mavis admired him for his perseverance and honesty, but he and Mattie were not being models of domestic tranquillity. Rumors spread that Brady had danced with another woman in a night club. Mavis tearfully related, "There was little joy in the home because rumors of my father being involved in an extra-marital affair cast jealousy and bitterness between them. Although based only on gossip, the situation was, to me, the most distressing and disastrous that could occur. Again I turned to God in my need, but my search for His leadership and comfort was outside the church." Mavis talked to her parents but felt her attempt had failed.[11]

In February of 1945, during Mavis's senior year of nurses' training, Brady came home early one morning after working the night shift. He milked the cows, walked into the house, went upstairs, and fell asleep. Suddenly, Mattie heard him shout. By the time she reached him he was dead, apparently from a massive heart attack.

Mavis was shattered. "Daddy died suddenly following the heart attack. . . to this day, the anguish of the loss of my father seems to be intensified by the unhappiness that existed between him and mother at the time."[12] The trauma of his death caused Mavis to ask questions. "I struggled, thinking my own power sufficient, not willing to seek God's full power and grace."[13]

Her dad's unexpected death did not deter Mavis from finishing nursing school. In a letter of recommendation, Dr. C. E. Boyd, chairman of the board of the Doctor's Hospital, wrote, "Miss Mavis O. Pate was graduated from the North Louisiana School of Nursing on August 31, 1945. She attended this school three years. To my personal knowledge, she was an excellent student, ranking high in her class, and graduated with the full respect of the entire faculty and of her classmates."[14] But how long would it be before Mavis would seek the Lord whose fellowship she apparently lost?

"Ankle Bill"

Following graduation from nursing school, Mavis began work at the C. E. Boyd Clinic and the North Louisiana Sanitarium. She enjoyed being close to Gwen who also was on the staff.

Mavis and Gwen roomed at the "Amos Rooming and Boarding House" in Shreveport until Gwen's marriage. They lived in a family setting with Widow Amos. Mavis valued her closeness to the family and her status as their "red-headed stepchild." Her example inspired Mrs. Amos's granddaughter later to become a nurse.

During this time Mavis began to question her faith. She felt that Protestant churches did not have their doctrine well defined. For a time the order and ritual of the Catholic Church challenged her. She talked to a priest and several preachers about her indecision. Her searching soon ended in an unexpected way.

World War II had ended, and the servicemen returned from Europe. Her U.S.O. boyfriend kept his promise and sought out Mavis. She reacted with ambivalence. "Actually, I wanted to be able to love him enough to marry him but did not find it possible. I hurt him deeply in not being able to accept the love offered . . . that was one of the most difficult moments in my life."[15]

The happy arrival of her sister Gwen's first child overshadowed her unhappiness. Joseph Brady Lewis was born on November 27, 1946. Mavis arranged to be on private duty for the delivery. "Little Joe" had a long and difficult delivery, and his head was ugly and elongated. But for Mavis he was the most beautiful baby in the world! When he finally arrived, Mavis ran out into the waiting room and announced to the family, "It's a boy. I'm an uncle!" One of Mavis's uncles earlier nicknamed her "Bill." So, her nieces and nephews called her "Ankle [sic] Bill" from this time on. She made it a habit of signing her family letters with the nickname "Bill."

Gwen soon moved to Arkansas with her new family, and Mavis moved to El Paso, Texas, to do her specialty as an operating-room nurse. She felt a camaraderie with the operating-room nurses. She moved so many places during this time that her family began calling her the "six-month girl."

Her first experience with people of a different culture unfolded when she trained at the Polyclinical Medical School and Hospital in New York City in 1948. She shared an apartment with four girls from the Philippines. Later she reflected that this experience "had a specific influence on my attitudes and prejudices in both group and personal relationships."[16] This later figured heavily in a pivotal decision in her life.

A new and positive change occurred in Mavis's family. Her mother, after several years of being a widow, married Johny Oden on July 29, 1948. In the exchange of vows, Mavis acquired a new brother and sister, Johny Hoyt and Genie Oden. Genie was only sixteen. Her mother died a year earlier. She and Mavis became close friends, and that association grew deeper in the future.

Mavis returned to home territory by this time and became assistant supervisor of the operating room at the Old Charity Hospital at Shreveport in 1949. Her experience in El Paso and New York had increased her competence in operating-room techniques. However, her efficiency and conscientiousness soon caused her problems. Her supervisor did not appreciate all of her expertise and her straightforward manner. Neither did she care for the recognition Mavis received from the doctors! So, in 1950 Mavis decided to make a move because of a "minor dispute with the supervisor." Charity offered her a scholarship to Northwestern State College to receive her B.S. degree in nursing on condition that she return and work at Charity for one year following graduation. Mavis returned to Old Charity Hospital to become operating-room supervisor. Mavis took charge of planning and equipping the new operating room.

Mavis found a new friend and confidant in her stepsister, Genie. In 1949 Genie married Van Norman and moved to Minden, Louisiana. Mavis visited Genie often to escape hospital responsibilities. Genie was involved in the Baptist Church in Minden, and missions was a real concern for her. This concern soon influenced Mavis.

Her studies and experience finally paid dividends. Mavis received her B.S. in Nursing at Northwestern State College in Natchitoches, Louisiana, in February 1952. She graduated with honors, having made twenty-two A's and only one B. She achieved academic and professional status and found herself at the top of the nursing profession. But there was still a strange sense of dissatisfaction in her heart.

"The Search"—Social Springs

After a season of spiritual wandering, Mavis returned to her own church to dig deeper into her faith. She sought a sign that she was on the right path. She wanted to hear a voice in the dark. Her life had to be "black and white and no gray," not only medically speaking, but also in the spiritual realm. Long talks with Genie began to take effect. The influence of Vivian Patterson, a nurse friend and dedicated Christian from Spring Hill, also deepened her own peace and faith in God.[17]

The turning point in Mavis's spiritual search came in 1953. She attended a revival meeting at Social Springs Baptist Church. She re-dedicated her life to Christ. There began a slow change in her attitude that had a decisive influence on her future.

This change became apparent when "J. D.," a medical salesman, invited her out. Mavis discovered that he was married but separated from his wife. She politely refused the date. "J. D." didn't give up. He was to figure in her life in later years.

One of Mavis's satisfying accomplishments in 1954 was the new design of an instrument tray. Her design simplified the handling of instruments during an operating procedure. The tray featured pegs that held the instruments open during the sterilization process, enabling the surgical staff to pick up all the instruments together and making them much easier to handle during operations. She sold the patent to the Ethicon Corporation.

Christian growth for Mavis was arduous. She received some satisfaction by singing the *Messiah* in a church choir. But a call to move to Tyler, Texas, in 1956 to become the operating-room supervisor at the Tyler Medical Center brought unexpected renewal in her spiritual life.

The Rose Capital

Mavis became active in the First Baptist Church of Tyler. Her Sunday School teacher, George Pearson, made a strong impression on her because of the "unaffected and deep Christian quality of his character." An even deeper impact was felt from the preaching and counseling of Dr. William Shamburger, pastor of the church. She later reflected, "I attribute much of my spiritual awakening, growth, and development to the stimulating preaching and leadership of this man of God."[18] Pastor Shamburger remembers Mavis fondly:[19]

Mavis Pate was a most gifted and dedicated young lady. She excelled in the quality of professional services she rendered in the operating rooms of the Medical Center Hospital, Tyler. She had a unique ability to relate to both the physicians and to the other nurses in that setting, and proved her skills daily in meeting the needs of each situation.

Though her work was heavily scheduled at the hospital, she always found time to faithfully attend the services and the ministries of First Baptist Church. She was much more than a mere "attender." She was a "contributor" to each facet of the church life in which she was involved. She demonstrated again and again her sensitivity to the feelings and needs of everyone around her.

Mavis lived in a trailer park. There she met a divorced man with a child. His curiosity about how much money she made aroused her suspicions. In her confusion she turned to her sister Gwen and to her mother and stepfather for advice. They felt the man wanted to use Mavis. Gwen told her, "If you marry him, you're marrying to support him." She accepted Gwen's advice but not without pain.

The ending of the relationship left Mavis in a deep emotional turmoil. It had a shaking effect that paid spiritual dividends. Mavis reflected, "I look back on that time as the first true and total realization of my own inadequacies and my need for Jesus as a personal Savior rather than a moral teacher."[20]

Through it all, Mavis never lost her uniqueness as a person, especially in the eyes of her younger relatives. They admired her unique life-style. Gwen's daughter, Pam, related:[21]

"Mavis was something different in the family. She was single, lived in a trailer, drove a white Studebaker Champion sports car, and took a lot of time with us kids. She would swoop in with her dog, always late, having driven all the way from Tyler. But we would always wait up until she got here. Mavis was a non-conformist. She would wear a white pump and a brown one. She liked not to be the same as everybody else. She was not exactly rebellious, but she was an individualist.

"Her dog, 'Duke,' was a little white thing with spots. She treated him like her child. Somebody poisoned 'Duke' with strychnine in 1956. We drove faster than I have ever been in a car—seventy-five or eighty miles an hour to Spring Hill to the vet. He gave the dog so many shots he stayed asleep for forty-eight hours. She put him in a box, and the dog howled until she took him out again.

"That dog could jump higher than any other dog! Whenever she opened the window of the car he could jump in or out. She took him to work with her and the dog would stay under the car in the parking lot. In Tyler the butcher would feed him every day. 'Duke' was everybody's friend.

"Mavis was strict with us kids. She treated us like her own. She used to smoke and drink beer in front of us, but she changed when she decided to go to seminary. She was different, exciting!"

Once again J. D. stepped back into her life. It was 1959, and his wife had died. Was Mavis interested now? Again came the response, "Once again in my life I felt guilty not being in love with one who apparently loved me."[22] An unexpected newspaper advertisement put this disappointment behind her.

"Project Hope" advertised for interested medical personnel to join the maiden voyage of the goodwill ship, the *S.S. Hope* to Southeast Asia in 1960. The idea intrigued Mavis. *Could this be the opportunity I have been waiting for?* she wondered. She talked with her trusted pastor, Dr. Shamburger. His response was, "The Lord always works in strange ways to lead us into His will. This experience may be the tool."[23] So she went for it! To her delight Project Hope accepted her as an operating-room nurse.

Mavis received a leave of absence from the Tyler Medical Center and left Duke with her mother. Mattie and Johnnie Oden drove Mavis west to San Francisco to meet the ship. After she arrived she learned to her surprise that she had been appointed as the operating-room supervisor for the *S.S. Hope*. Also, the Ethicon Corporation, one of the major project sponsors, asked her to write a diary of the voyage.

Her expertise as a writer had become known through the publication of her article on "Orienting the Student of X-Ray Technology to the Operating Suite" (in the September 1959 issue of *Operating Room Digest*). The adventure on the *S.S. Hope* would radically alter the direction of her life!

3

Voyage on the *Ship Hope*

The *Ringgold Record* of Friday, July 1, 1960, carried the following lead article about Mavis;

MISS MAVIS PATE TO GO ON
MEDICAL EXPEDITION TO ASIA

Miss Mavis Pate, a former Ringgold resident, will be one of 22 nurses selected from over 1,000 applicants to take part in Project 'HOPE' (Health Opportunity for People Everywhere), a part of the government's People to People program.

The project will take Miss Pate on a year-long medical expedition to Indonesia and Viet Nam.

Miss Pate, the daughter of Mrs. Johnnie H. Oden, now lives at Tyler, Texas. She was valedictorian of the Class of 1942 at Ringgold High School. She is a graduate of the North Louisiana Sanitarium School of Nursing and Northwestern State College. . . .

Miss Pate explains that Project HOPE is a part of the People to People Health Foundation which is private, independent and non-profit and was formed to carry out a cooperative health program between the people of the United States and those in friendly countries abroad. However, it will only enter a country when invited by the medical profession of that country.

The ship will be operated free by the American President Lines and will serve as a medical school, a training and treatment center, and a base for medical, nursing, and sanitation teams. It will also be the logistics center for medical aid and health exchange programs. In emergencies the ship has 800 beds but for the trip only about 268 will be utilized. It will be staffed with 15 doctors, 22 nurses, two dentists and various technical and administrative personnel. Total costs for a year's operation will be about $3,000,000.

Although Miss Pate does not know what her specific duties will be, she knows that the method of operation will include two teams. One of the teams will stay on the ship most of the time and teach classes in the various phases of medicine. They will train native workers. The other half will go ashore and teach and treat. The work will be directed toward nurses and technicians . . . instead of at doctors because a large mass can be reached.

Mavis documented her voyage on the *S.S. Hope* by regular letters home to her family. They are treasures to be shared.

Wed. Sept. 21, 1960
On Board *S.S. Hope*
The days have been filled with fascinating and different things. For example, I was just interrupted in the first sentence of this epistle to appear on the helicopter decks in a bathing suit for publicity pictures of the swimming pool (portable type) that was just brought aboard. Now I am waiting for the bells to ring for a fire drill . . .

Wednesday, Sept. 14, 1960—It was necessary for me to complete my Merchant Marine and Coast Guard papers . . . I was "sworn in" as an Ordinary Seaman, and I carry a card to say so.

Thursday, Sept. 15, 1960—Sandwiched in a bit of last-minute shopping and sightseeing. We will have one more chance to decide what else we have forgotten and to pick it up in Hawaii. Rah!

Friday, Sept. 16—Read this week's *Life* magazine for words and pictures describing this day. And the mops and brooms are not just for publicity. We use them from about 10 A.M. until 4:30 P.M. and briskly too. There are three operating rooms in my department. We made a Fibber McGee closet out of two of them, stacking cartons, furniture, etc., and one we cleared out decently enough for Open House. To date I have not seen any supplies or equipment for the department. Preparation and organization of supplies and instruments will keep us busy on the way to Indonesia. I have already imagined my helplessness if on the first day out one of the crew gets appendicitis and they turn to me and say, "How soon can you have a room ready to go?" Pocket knife, please!

Monday, Sept. 19—We moved on board the ship and signed "on" for the voyage. Quite a procedure. And, at last, I had all suitcases, trunk, and boxes in one place. My stateroom is very nice, adequate room, comfortable and I have two roommates . . . no complaints here. Confusion is running rampant at the moment. All family and friends are on board for Bon Voyage. Excitement is contagious and all have a share to give away.

Wednesday, Sept. 21—The officials of Ethicon were here at noon to discuss the articles that I am to attempt to write while away. They are making it extremely convenient for me. They presented me with a tape recorder (tapes of music included—Oh Boy!) and a camera. I am thrilled over the opportunity this is going to be but again wonder at my ability to give them what they can print.

And briefly that brings you up to date. Oh, there are oodles of little exciting details (like "to the helicopter deck in full uniform with cap" for pictures to be shot from a helicopter overhead!).

Everybody use that address,

Mavis, alias "Ankle Bill"

Wednesday Night, Sept. 28, 1960—On Board the Hope
And I didn't get seasick. In fact, only two or three of the entire group had any trouble at all.

I was very proud of "my crew" and thought that things went as smoothly as clockwork. We have had our test and proved that we can function—we're over the first hump.

There are many more interesting details and sidelights that I wish I could tell but time does not permit. One thing, however, I must tell briefly. We have had exceptionally good lectures since leaving San Francisco. Mr. Galbraith of the Department of State and Mr. Good-friend, the author of *Rice Roots,* have lectured from 1-4 P.M. and 7-9 P.M. each day. They have presented some of the political, social, and cultural background of the Indonesian people which has been most interesting and will be most helpful.

More from Djakarta . . .

Love you all, Bill

"Shellback"

The Ethicon Corporation sent the following letter to Mavis's family.
It describes the unforgettable event of *crossing the equator*, a stopover
in Balikpapan, and includes some personal notes to the family:
October 15th was a red letter day in the voyage from Honolulu to
Djakarta. This was the day we passed over the equator. You doubtless
have heard of the initiation ceremonies that change one into a shell-
back once he has passed the equator. This particularly holds true on
board ship. To have flown over the equator is not quite the same. Now
I understand why, because how could they have such an initiation
ceremony aboard a plane? Our initiation began about 7:30 A.M.
Those who had crossed the equator, known as shellbacks, planned the
afternoon for the polywogs, that is, the uninitiated. The ceremonies
began on the helicopter deck. We were duly introduced to King Neptune and his court. Following this was a reception—if one wishes to
call it that—in the ward recreation room. There was a judging of the
nautical costumes which were worn to the initiation ceremony. It was a
big evening for the personnel and crew alike. Great fun for all!

On Sunday, October 16th, a day after King Neptune's party and
after we were all initiated as shellbacks, we arrived in Balikpapan.
That is a port in Borneo. The stop in Balikpapan was for refueling
only. However, we had several hours there—long enough for us to
take a short trip into the city and see some of the local color. The
Balikpapan branch of the Shell Oil Company provided transportation
and made this trip possible.

Sailing time from Balikpapan presented something typical of the
philosophy of the people of this part of the world. Sailing time had
been set for 6 o'clock and at that time we learned that the Indonesian
customs had not returned the ship's papers. So, sailing was delayed
about one hour. They never seem to be in a hurry here. There's another custom which I think we might take advantage of—that is an afternoon siesta. I can see it now—stop surgery, go to lunch, and we'll take
a one-hour siesta.

Now a personal note . . .

There are many things I miss, like the old Studebaker and my good ol' hound dog and the peace and quiet of the countryside. These things I am sure I will appreciate a great deal more when I return.

Wednesday in Surabaja, November 9, 1960
Dear Friends and Family of the Hopeless Nurse of *Hope*,
I have succumbed to the seagoing hazard of losing all sense of time. I can no longer keep track of what month, day, or time of day it is. The funny thing is that you turn to the next fellow and ask him and he is no more sure than you are. Therein lies part of my excuse for infrequent reports and the lack of continuity of the ones I make.

That last little epistle which I imposed on Ethicon to send out for me was quite a one! My state of mind was such that I'm sure whatever I wrote did not make much sense. The week in Djakarta taxed my mental and physical strength as much as any week I have ever spent. There was no major incident accounting for this, just many and varied small things . . .

We sailed from Djakarta about 10 A.M. on the 2nd of November— At any rate, the two days at sea were a welcome relief for all. We arrived in Surabaja at about 9 A.M. on the 4th. Working time (during those two sailing days and for the first two days after arrival) was spent in regrouping the forces and "shaping things up." Patients are not admitted the first two days in port. The doctors aboard visited the local hospitals and selected the patients for admission.

The first patients were admitted on Monday, Nov. 7 and our first surgery was scheduled on Tuesday. They assigned two more American nurses to the operating room and central supply department and we have four Indonesian nurses on a six-month status.

There are such differences as . . . Have you ever tried to tell an orderly to go to the laundry, take the dirty linen and pick up the clean linen when neither party involved can understand or speak more than a dozen words of the other's language (and those dozen words are not the ones you need for that particular conversation)? Or better still, direct him to disinfect a room when not only does he not understand the language but even if he did, he cannot fathom the need for cleaning a room when he can't "see" any dirt there to begin with. Then it is interesting to instruct nurses in your way of doing things without the benefit of the spoken word.

By finagling out of that one (a program at the university med school in Surabaja) I have to attend a dinner at the American Consulate next Tuesday. At least it is an eating meeting! There is an activity I am anticipating with a little more pleasure tomorrow night. The ship's officers and medical crew are invited to a dance at the local Navy Officer's Club. I will get to wear my lace overskirt.

This must suffice for this time. I am being forbidden to partake of the coffee until I finish this so I can see nothing else to do but discontinue at this point. See, what did I tell you? It is so easy to procrastinate when distractions are so close.

Love and Miss you All

Bill

In Surabaja, Indonesia, Mavis visited a place which would have a decisive influence on her life and future:

Monday, Nov. 14, 1960

Two Surabajan nurses were to come on at 7 A.M. but were not here so I think they have changed them to come on at 8 A.M. There was scuttlebut (gossip) to that effect and that is the best communication that one gets. Then on the way back from that dry-run the little Indonesian elevator boy stopped me to show me that he had knocked the nail off his big toe! . . . The best part of the day was at the end when my Indonesian aides or orderlies disappeared about 3:15 without bringing up the clean linen and I don't know if they still don't understand these things or need to be relieved of the position.

Tuesday, Nov. 15, 1960

Woke up this A.M. with the "native malady." We were to attend a dinner at the home of the American consul, the one social obligation which I was anticipating with pleasure and I'm home on a liquid diet— The second day of the malady threw me all off schedule and here it is Nov. 29 and I'm not back on schedule yet. The "native malady" is nothing to worry about, just what we would call intestinal virus at home. The people here have been very friendly and receptive in every way. I visited in one of the Indonesian nurse's home and had a very pleasant time.

I had the experience of a lifetime this weekend. I visited a Southern Baptist Mission Hospital. It is located in Kediri, a small town about midway between this coastline of Java and the southern coastline. I would guess it is about 100 to 115 miles from Surabaja. The hospital is one of the best I have seen (or heard about) in Indonesia and it was an inspiration to meet the people there. They were all Southerners besides being Southern Baptist. The pioneer in the establishment and building of the hospital is a woman doctor, Dr. Kathleen Jones, who had gone to Dallas Medical School and knew many of the Tyler doctors. She is one of the finest people! This was sort of a *Hope* Mission trip. I went up with two of the doctors and another nurse from the ship . . . We spent the night there, and did two surgery procedures. My biggest regret was that it rained all the time and I'm afraid I will not have any pictures.

The visit to the Baptist Hospital in Kediri apparently planted a spiritual seed in Mavis's heart that bore fruit in a commitment to missions in the future. But her life-style required some definite changes. Devout Southern Baptists are still a socially conservative people. Most abstain from drinking alcoholic beverages. Smoking is frowned upon by many. The language used by some O. R. nurses is unacceptable in Baptist missionary circles! Any change is Mavis's habits would wait for a later time, as we see from her letters from *Bali, Indonesia:*

Tues. Dec. 6, 1960
We are now anchored off the shore of the fantabulous isle of Bali, and it is almost as beautiful and exotic as the movies and storybooks would have you believe! Since we could not dock, bringing patients on board the ship is a problem so the local committee sent in teams to the four hospitals to do their work there. Can you imagine 15 doctors, 4 hospitals, 1,800,000 people and trying to do something of lasting consequence in less than three weeks? . . .

You would never guess in a hundred years what I'm doing at the moment— sitting at the vanity drinking a bourbon (of which Chuck

probably will not approve) with a Beauty Counselor pack on my face
and my feet soaking in a basin of chlorine water.

Dec. 15, 1960

I continuously search the English language for words to adequately
portray my surroundings, my experiences, and my thoughts . . . One
should have an instantaneous telepathy recorder to record one's
thoughts and reactions to each new sight and experience and could be
mailed home. . . .

With overnight bag for a day or two on location and a box or two of
instruments and sutures, plus all cameras just like tourists, it is a neat
trick to catch the ship on the down swell and the launch on the up
swell and not end up somewhere in between. The twenty minutes of
boating over are very pleasant with the gentle sea swells, a cool sea
breeze, brilliant blue water, a beautiful mountainous shoreline with
Bali High peeking out over a cloud, and Lombok and other small islands visible on the horizon to the left. Then we make the landing at
Pandangbay!

There is always a crowd of small children to welcome us. Children
are children all over the world, bright-eyed, uninhibited, curious, and
happy. All of them have learned at least one English word, "Hello,"
and can carry on a whole conversation with it. Most of them are very
healthy, robust looking, and some of the 10-year-olds can carry a load
that would slow me down considerably.

We go to the Customs Office to register the cameras and locate the
bus— Everyone gets settled on whatever the transportation may be
and when the driver (always Indonesian because I don't think anyone
else could maneuver the wrong side of the road, European style,
around all the bicycles, pony carts, pigs, chickens, women with loads
on their heads, and men with balanced shoulder yoke loads) decides to
show up, we begin the 1 hour and 45 minute drive. Nature and her
beauty are enough to keep one enthralled for the entire drive even if
one did not find the individuals and local culture so fascinating. Vegetation is of the lush, green, tropical type one would expect. And
though it is abundant, it is not dense or impenetrable looking. There
are coconut palms, banana trees, banyan trees, and then those which I
do not know. And, though the rice paddies are not natural, they are so

arranged to utilize nature and her forces until one begins to consider them a product of nature. Truly the layouts and irrigation systems are a stroke of engineering genius amidst the existing dearth of mechanical development. Besides all this, they make a beautiful landscape in symmetry and color.

We see many activities of everyday life along the roadside. Women do much of the heavy work, and you see practically all of them engaged in some task while a large percentage of the men appear to be idle. Ninety-five percent of the women that you see walking along are carrying something on their heads, but you never see a man carrying anything on his head. If he has a load to carry, he carries it on a double-yoke-like thing similar to balance scales. I saw a real gentleman the other day. He was assisting the lady in getting her 50-pound basket up on her head! And I saw a woman blacktopping the street in Denpasar.

Other activities frequently noted are the tending of the duck flocks. A man with a long staff of bamboo, a flag tied on it, and a flock of 50 to 75 ducks all in very orderly fashion close by, or if it is meal time the tender will stick the staff into the ground and depart from the field but the ducks remain close by the staff. The ducks are used similarly to geese in the States to eat undesirable vegetation out of the desirable crop, in this instance, rice. Farmers cultivate the wet rice field by walking or tromping in it barefooted; spreading of sea water on the salt flats or salt troughs for evaporation thereby producing salt (all table salt here is very coarse and unsalty, reminds me of "hominy snow"); gathering mature rice, a process reminiscent of cutting flowers stem by stem; beating rice into flour with a wooden bowl and mortar; sewing done by men. They do have sewing machines and I did see a woman sewing in the market the other day—markets in a similar fashion to French Market in New Orleans with open stalls and a little of everything that is to be bought—and what sewing I have seen is very crude; soccer games by the children and teenagers; men pruning and petting their favorite fighting cock; basket weaving; and then there are many just sitting! Someone made the statement the other day that we probably spend as much time in front of the television but the Indonesian just takes a seat on the side of road and sees quite a show.

Bicycles (*the* mode of transportation), pigs, cows, and chickens frequently demand their share of the road. Driving is done by the use of the horn in all parts of Indonesia . . . A drive through either town or country is heralded by the almost constant sound of the horn . . . In Djakarta and Surabaja, the two larger cities of Java, the *boetchek* is the way to travel. The boetchek is a bicycle with a two-wheeled seat for two attached in front. It is a leisurely and quite pleasant way to travel, like a slow roadster with the top down—fascinating on a South Pacific, moonlit night. Here on the island of Bali, it is not considered equal to a man's dignity to pedal people in a boetchek, so they have pony carts. The ponies are very small, like a Shetland pony, and boy can they singlefoot! The cart has a top like the surrey with the fringe.

We took a pony cart out to one of the two hospitals in Denpasar. Let it suffice to say that in many respects, the conditions are deplorable. There is a drastic shortage of equipment, supplies, drugs, organizational know-how, and doctors. There is no shortage of nurses, but there is a shortage of nursing care and nursing knowledge. However, I feel that the entire medical team (Indonesian) deserves commendation for being able to function at all under such adverse conditions. We, who are accustomed to more, would think that we could not.

Since we are anchored out at sea, bringing patients on board has presented some additional problems . . . they must be ambulatory both when admitted and when discharged. However, we have a high census of 36 patients on board now and would be doing some surgery each day but for the lack of blood. We are doing a considerable amount of chest X-Rays on board the ship, as many as can be transported out and run through the mill. We have one of the Rajah's nine wives on board as a patient and a second one with her to keep her company because she got lonesome.

Monday, Dec. 26, 1960—Bali, Indonesia
HAPPY NEW YEAR, ALL!!
CHRISTMAS and NEW YEAR in Bali are different from any heretofore, I must say! The holidays aboard *S.S. Hope* have been wonderful, actually, with real trees, real Christmas decorations, and real Christmas wrapped packages. There is something lacking though—that Christmas Spirit!

Yesterday was quite a full day. Got up at 6:30 (yes I did!) for Protestant Communion Services, breakfasted at 8:10, gift exchange followed. Then Protestant Services at 9:00, Tom & Jerry party at 10:00 and then left on a boating excursion at 11:00. The Chief Engineer arranged to use the Captain's Gig (lifeboat and roustabout) and 12 of us took a long cruise down the island shoreline. We anchored and went swimming off the side. Then the rains came! Just like spring showers! Another thing not like the Christmas season, my first sunburn of the whole voyage on Christmas Day! The rain brought us back to the ship earlier than planned, before the large dinner.

All of the Indonesian nurses and doctors entered into the activities wholeheartedly. In fact we have several Christians among those sailing with us and I'm sure we had many visitors at the Christmas services. The Medical Staff drew names together, doctors and nurses, Indonesian and American, and then my five girls in the O.R. gave me individual gifts. It was very sweet and considerate of them but it made me feel badly, because they have so very little as it is.

Jan. 20, 1961—Makasar, Indonesia

I'm sure whatever the year with HOPE brings, it will be new, different, and a challenge . . . Challenges such as a water leak in the ceiling directly over the OR table with an operation in progress, the OR floor flooded by a "busted" fire hose when you arrive to begin a morning schedule, finding that Scotch bottles work nicely as disinfectant solution bottles, making cleft lip splints out of steinman pins, and borrowing vice grip and plain pliers and hacksaw from the engineers for an intramedullary nailing. Never a dull moment!

The rebel action differs here also. There is more of it. Of course, we don't see anything except the gunshot wounds in the hospitals, but there are allusions to it all the time.

Back to the lack of things, it is almost impossible to get donors for blood in this area. We were told this was because most of the people hold to the superstition that if they give blood to another person, they give their power to that person. . . . We finally received some long-awaited supplies today . . . it was a very disappointing delivery . . . the supplies arrived in very poor shape. Most of the foodstuffs had been

ruined by water and many, many crates had been torn into and
pilfered.

Feb. 8, 1961—Makasar, Indonesia

We are all getting as bad as the saltiest sailor. We look forward to
setting sail for a new port. The time at sea is very restful and refreshing after three weeks of looking from the inside to the outside of the
human zoo.

In addition to that, I would have missed the burial at sea. Sound
morbid don't I, but it is something that I probably will never experience again. One of the crew members expired aboard ship about two
weeks ago. He was Chief Boatswain. In view of the fact that he had not
listed a single relative or next of kin on any of his official papers and
none could be located, he is to be buried at sea. This has to be done in
International Waters according to the "code of the sea," therefore, the
ceremony will be held while we are enroute to Ambon.

March 3, 1961—Ambon, Indonesia

Have had a crisis develop . . . a mild wind and rainstorm. The ship
is not very rough but small craft were having a difficult time about 30
minutes ago. As the Indonesian launch was preparing to leave from
shore to make a trip out to *Hope*, some man on the dock got caught
between two boats and got a crushed leg.

The crisis just previous to this one was the saddest to all of us. One
of the lab technicians, Lois Boyce, started having headaches and other
vague difficulties. As things developed, they suspected a brain tumor
and arranged with the American Embassy to have a plane fly her to
the Air Force Hospital in Japan. This was Feb. 24. Lois was operated
on for the brain tumor in Japan and expired two days Post-op. A very
sad situation.

One half of the year is gone. In a way I can hardly believe it and in
another it seems as though it has been forever. I am looking forward to
the next six months, particularly visiting Singapore and the possibility
of taking my vacation in Hong Kong.

March 5, 1961, Sunday P.M.—Ambon, Indonesia

The beach party for the surgery crew did proceed as planned yesterday. The ten-mile drive out was interesting and picturesque. It began
by one driver knocking down a poor defenseless little kid-goat which

sounded like a child crying as it lay in the street. The trip progressed out of the town along narrow, partially asphalt roads, past numerous bamboo-thatch dwellings. Invariably, these houses have a small but immaculately kept yard, swept as clean as the palm of your hand. There is as (a general rule) no semblance of closures for the windows or doors other than a piece of batik hanging over them. And it always seems that when vehicles such as ours pass, someone has sent the word ahead. Men, women, and children are standing alongside the road to watch us go by. Most of the time, they are expressionless . . . but at the first expression of greeting on our part, they flash a wide smile and wave in the friendliest manner. Children, in groups, as at school or at play, will yell, dance around, and wave even before we greet them. However there are a few, such as a couple of 9 or 10-year-old boys who did not greet us and when we waved to them, they frowned and spit in our direction. This response is only a small minority and is far outweighed by the friendly response usually encountered.

The water was beautiful and clear, the bottom rather rocky and filled with coral which makes it very picturesque and interesting for snorkeling. We were watching the Indonesian custom (and ability) to dress in a mixed group by using the sarong. It is quite an interesting and intriguing art to hold the sack-like creation, about a yard and one-half in circumference, on the shoulders and in the mouth and put on one's clothes underneath without the least bit of exposure. This is an art the Indonesians develop in the process of bathing in the rivers or streams which are not only visible for all passersby, but they are also co-educational. Usually they are divided so that the man and boys utilize the river on the left side of the bridge and the women and girls on the right side, if there happens to be a bridge.

(Mavis usually enjoyed life, but the reality of death is never far away for an operating-room nurse. To a degree, it curbed her "uninhibited expression of joy in life." Death came from time to time to the crew of the Hope.) Mavis included the following in her letters home.

ORDER OF EVENTS FOR THE *BURIAL AT SEA*
OF BOS'N JOHN R. O'MEARA

0800—Prepare helicopter deck. Remove chairs, sweep down, prepare platform, shroud and flowers.

0930—Deck Honor Guard remove Bos'n O'Meara from hospital area to helicopter deck making ready for burial, covering body with flag.

0945—All hands assemble in areas designated on plan. Uniform: Officers—dress whites; Medical—uniform; Deck and Engine Crew—dungarees and white "T" shirts; Quartermasters—khakis; Stewards—white trousers and jackets.

1000—Stop engines. Flag half-masted at gaff. Father Magner officiates and when finished Honor Guard consigns body to deep. At that time, Captain will give order for right-hand salute.

Delegates then drop flowers on sea, and salute completed. Assembly dismissed, flag two blocked. Resume course and speed.

All hands are requested not to take cameras to the ceremony. Arrangements have been made with the ship's photographer to take the required pictures for official purposes and for Bos'n O'Meara's shipmates.

The same letter of Sunday March 6, 1961 included this humorous allusion to her friend Chuck.

I will admit to you that I spend a great deal of my spare time in pursuit of personal interests . . . that is my interest in the engineering department. But then you know that I have always been sort of mechanically inclined. Ha!

(The *Hope* continued its voyage through the islands of Indonesia. One island, Timor, later became famous through the book, *Like a Mighty Wind,* by Mel Tari who described a spiritual renewal among the local people.)[1]

Tuesday, March 7, 1961

If you recall, white is one of my favorite colors but I restrained myself and did not bring more than 25 or 30 pieces in white and then we have six white uniforms. Had, I should say! We have two kinds of water problems. Not only the shortage mentioned before but all the storage tanks have reached the stage of iron oxidation! Now we have beige underclothes, blouses, uniforms, etc. Oh well, who wants white clothes anyway?

Thursday, March 9, 1961

I am going to have a complaint to voice when I get home. I do not get the opportunities that the Indonesian OR Supervisor does. He is a male montrie (which falls in the medical classification somewhere between a doctor and a nurse). He not only administers the department but also does some minor surgery. For example, the Island of Timor did not have a doctor from Jan. 1960 when the Dutch doctor was forced to leave until 3 months ago when a Chinese doctor came. The male montrie did what was done in the way of surgery in the meantime, mostly lacerations and that sort of thing.

Saturday, March 11, 1961

There are some native dances scheduled tonight for our benefit so I'll put on my bib and tucker and go. They staged it very nicely, had a raised stage at one end of the Gunung Juanita (translated means Woman's Building) with a drawn curtain and potted palm trees on the backdrop. The music was live instruments and vocal. They have one instrument that is peculiar to this island only. It is a stringed instrument, roughly one piece of bamboo log about 2 ft. long resting inside ½ bamboo log slightly larger with the strings stretched the length of the thing in between the two. Sounds similar to an extremely high-pitched guitar.

Friday, March 17, 1961

The Moslem faction of the Indonesian personnel aboard celebrated the end of their month's fasting (they neither eat nor drink from sunrise until sunset during the month) with a feast and entertainment to which they invited the entire ship's compliment. There were oodles of Indonesian food, which I can best describe as resembling Chinese food, not quite so tasty, but somewhat warm with peppers, Indonesian music, and Indonesian dances.

Wednesday, March 22, 1961

Did 14 cases ranging from thyroidectomy to local T. & A.

Thursday, March 23, 1961

A surgeon saw a patient in the clinic with bladder carcinoma. He felt that a resection of this tumor would give the patient at least five more years of life . . . was advised that the equipment be taken ashore and the procedure be accomplished there. Three problems—getting machine onto launch, out of launch onto jetty, from jetty to jeep, and thus to hospital. This is not a usual responsibility of the urological surgeon but it helps build up the muscles, and after all, there are no golf courses in Indonesia.

Monday, March 27, 1961
An earthquake had been reported on the island of Flores. Arrived at the entrance of the Bay of Ende this A.M. about 7. A survey team went ashore to see what the situation was. Returning about 11:30 the group reported that at one time the hospital was fairly full of slightly injured victims but most had gone because of fear of additional earthquakes. There was about 50% destruction of those buildings damaged.

Wednesday, March 29, 1961
Arrived at Bima Harbor a little ahead of expected time of arrival. As we entered, there was a little boat on its way out of the harbor. Turned out that it contained the mayor, the one doctor, customs official and one other dignitary. They were on their way out of the harbor to go shark fishing. Boy, were they surprised!

Sunday, April 2, 1961
Easter sunrise services held on sun deck at 6 A.M. but doesn't really seem like Easter. No new hat or shoes. Ha!

(It appears that Mavis, despite her efficiency and professional competence, managed to adapt to most of the unusual situations encountered aboard the Ship *Hope.* Except for one!)

Monday, April 10, 1961
They snitched my three orderlies to assist in the visitor program. Without so much as a by-your-leave! And I lost my temper! Can you imagine? My losing my temper?

Wednesday, April 12, 1961
We have anchored off Lombok at Ampanan. We will go ashore to set up polyclinic tomorrow and to screen the patients they have lined up for us. It seems that the patient load here is not going to be too heavy. Only 53 are on the pre-selected list for us to see. There are some factors which might attribute to this, among them that 90% of the people here are of the Moslem religion and do not believe in male doctors treating female patients. I understand the Commies are at work in several areas around here. In fact, we get the impression that

there are a few following us around trying to foul up the works for us, but it is very quiet and subtle—no immediate danger to us.

(On its next stop, the *Hope* encountered unexpected difficulty that strained the ingenuity of Mavis and the engineering department.)

May 18, 1961—Bandung, Indonesia

We had an entirely new and different experience during our sail from Lombok to Semarang. At three o'clock in the morning everyone (except yours truly) was awakened by noises and vibrations somewhat resembling a small earthquake. *The S.S. Hope had run aground on a coral reed* about 400 yards off the shore of Sapudi Island. About 1/3 of the front end of the ship was resting on the bottom. Immediate reversal of the engines did no good. Preparations were begun to lighten the front (bow, that is) by moving fuel oil to the tanks in the stern and by emptying the ballast tanks (filled with H^2O for stability). At about 9 a.m. (high morning tide) they attempted to pull it back again with the engines. Again not successful. It was announced that a final attempt would be made at 9:30 P.M. (high evening tide) and removal of weight was continued. The two bow anchors were put down and back about 1/3 of the way of the ship and rigged with runners to act as pulleys. The failure of this attempt would mean notifying Djakarta to send out tug boats to pull us off. This would have meant 5-7 days time sitting on the rock.

With all preparations made an hour or two before high tide, we sat back to wait. The odds were running high that we would not be able to pull ourselves off. Seems this is quite an uncommon feat, once a ship is aground. Me—I had faith in my boy, Chuck.

Sure enough, as soon as the tide rose enough and with the pull of the anchors, she started sliding off. The engines were started immediately and we were free. However, in the process of backing out, the propeller hit an obstruction and bent up the edges. As soon as the ship was in safe water—about 10:30 P.M.—the anchor was dropped to wait until morning. This was done so that the ballasting tanks could be refilled and stability restored more positively. With that done, we continued our journey to Semarang. Semarang knew nothing of why the delay until they heard it on the Voice of America broadcast. Radioed to San Francisco—to Washington *Hope* office—To Voice of America and back!!

(The stopover in Semarang frustrated Mavis. The ship anchored about five miles from shore and ship personnel commuted by boat and bus each day. The difference in working schedules between Indonesians and Americans suspended many of her lectures or cancelled operations.)

May 18, 1961, Bandung, Indonesia

I don't know what I would do if a bunch of goons moved into *my* OR, the way we are expected to do. All in all, everyone is very gracious and things go fairly smoothly.

Bandung is a lovely mountain city about 150 miles from Djakarta where a very progressive medical school and school of nursing are located.

Actually the ten nurse-teachers who were assigned to *Hope* for seven months were from the school. We did a little work there in the hospital and held some lectures. But we were all convinced that we were invited there in order that they might show off their most westernized city, most pleasant climate and the medical facilities, which were the best we had seen in all our travels.

(The final days in Indonesia were full of various formal "send-off" receptions with officials along with the usual hospital schedule. The farewell event touched Mavis despite her seeming willingness to leave.)

We had "graduation" exercises for the Indonesian nurses yesterday afternoon. They moved off the ship afterward and then came back this a.m. to see us off. There were tears and handshakes and address exchanges all over the place. And we steamed out of our last Indonesian harbor at 8:00 this morning. Can't say as I'm sorry at all. It was quite an experience but I'm glad it's over.

The Project Hope contribution to Indonesia received acclaim from the American Ambassador to Indonesia, Howard P. Jones (as reported in *News from The People to People Health Foundation, Inc.* June 5 1961:

To the Captain, men and women of the medical staff and ship's personnel of the *S.S. Hope*. As the *Hope* leaves Indonesian waters after almost eight months of its angel of mercy mission, I want to congratulate everyone who participated in this pioneer undertaking. You made a great contribution in literally bringing hope and healing to many. You won the hearts of the Indonesians as I know they won yours. On behalf of the American government I wish to express my deep appreciation to all of you. The spirit of Project Hope will remain in the hearts and minds of all of us here.

Hong Kong welcomed the *Hope* next. The ship dry-docked for repairs on the hull and propeller. It also afforded an ideal place for shopping while awaiting news of whether or not a trip could be scheduled to Saigon. War clouds formed over Southeast Asia.

June 10, 1961—Hong Kong, China

We arrived in Hong Kong at about 10 A.M. but it was after 2:00 P.M. before we were situated in the drydock and the gangplank was put down. Many were on the rail ready to ride the gangplank down with bags in hand. A large percentage of those left aboard went to hotels for the length of the stay here.

Finally, today, we learned that we definitely would go on to Saigon as planned. After the rest (if you are not careful how you use the term) in Hong Kong and the boost in morale that it has given us all, I am ready to try it again.

(Saigon proved to be a very modern city with little need of the medical expertise of the *Hope* staff. But it taught Mavis a lot.)

June 20, 1961—Saigon, Vietnam

By the way, none of us knows any Vietnamese and it is a most difficult language to learn. It is a very tonal language where one word means many things depending on the roll of the tongue. Even French is not too useful if one happened to know it. I'm for a universal language after this, and naturally it would be English!

I was not very interested in the clothes in Indonesia. The sarong just wasn't as intriguing as the movies made out. The other costumes of the various islands did not do a thing for me. But the native dress of the Viet Namese is different. I like it. It is a very simple and very graceful costume. They wear long satin trousers with a dress over them. The dress is made almost exactly like the Chinese choengsan except that it is split up to the waist line on each side. It will make a lovely lounging outfit for the U.S. (or if I ever have nerve enough to wear it anyplace else).

I went over to Cholon for dinner, which is the Chinese section of Saigon. The dinner was very good! Eight course real Chinese food. Was all very good but the Duck Paw soup was sorta poor psychologically. I could see the Duck Paw. Have learned to eat and like the Bedams (century eggs that are cured in potash, spices, and mud 'n stuff, and come out of it all black).

(Mavis welcomed the cruise back to U.S.A. The adventure on the Ship *Hope* had been long and filled with the unexpected.)

Sunday, August 13, 1961—Saigon, Vietnam

Our activity here has been so rushed that I am definitely looking forward to the twenty-one days it will take us to cross the Pacific. I have dreams of not going back to work until Nov. 1st but am thinking that it is only a dream. Work here has not been so fantastically different from day to day as previously. Not that it has been routine either—but the crises are becoming routine now. Boy, will I ever be glad to settle down to one set of surgeons for a year or two! Six weeks of one and then an entirely new one is quite trying. You never quite get one's routine settled, what with all the improvisions and substitutions until you have to start over again. And true to form, they can't settle for the same substitutes. Oh well—won't be much longer and besides, some of them have been great guys. And it has been a great challenge, but deliver me from challenges for a week or two!

(The local Vietnamese staff Mavis had trained appreciated her more than she realized. To her surprise she received the following poignant letters:)

Saigon, Vietnam, August, 1961

Dear Pate,

My name is Nguyeh-Van-Hop. I am very please, I was order of my principle's (sic) hospital, he send me go down to work at the Hope. I am very please to make you acquaintance and everybody at the operating room, but I am sorry that I don't speak English very well. So sometimes you speak I don't understand or I speak you don't understand. However during time I work, I was guide by you and everybody. So I gather very much result. But during time I work with you, if I make a mistaken you forgive me. Because we are separation. So before you and everybody return come back you national to go on you work, I hope that you try help for people and I believer that I see you again.

Before stop my pen I true bid you and everybody I know a good voyage and my kindest regard to you parents and same your family, you please give me your address, what number of your house and street. From time to time I can send letter for you. My address is Nguyen-Van-Hop's Hospital, Gia-dinh.

In this letter if I write a mistaken excuse me. Because my family very poor I have not money to learn. So now I begin learn English. I true thank you very much.

Sincerely,
Nguyen-Van-Hop

Saigon, August 2nd, 1961

My dear Pate,

It is my great pleasure when I write this letter to you. But from you go I often feel very sad, everyday coming to office and going into dissection room, and sometimes on my way home, your image always appears sweetly in my mind. And particularly when I see the supplies putting in the operation room at that moment, I remember Eye by Miss Pate, my considerable friend. And I still keep in my memory the tiredness, and the business after a hard days work; and the late evenings for ORC. All both we must be hungry. Why Miss Pate, this dissection room must stop its activity for a short time maybe two months; because there is no patients. The doctor there had to return his old position now and he doesn't know certainly when he came back here ORC. . . . Why Pate, I always trouble to think on your long journey and I often pray you is in good health after many days gliding over so many belows and the immense ocean.

Dear Pate my charming friend, when you come to your native country please write some letters to me, Pate and tell me about the beautiful sites of you loving USA country because this country is told that there stand many fashionable houses, magnificent buildings, many imposing monuments, and the immense and boundless fields, many meadows fields.

Pate allow me to stop here. Pate don't forget me! I wish you and your family get good health, and to peace, enjoy the lives full of happiness.

Nhu Lien

(The *S.S. Hope* arrived in San Francisco on September 13, 1961. Mavis recorded these humorous thoughts:)

As far as "Project Hope's" plans for shore activities in the next port of call, namely San Francisco, we have been given specific instructions to "play it by ear." I understand English is the national dialect, the rate of exchange is 100:1, food and water ashore is comparatively safe if you choose the establishment carefully. There are dry-cleaning services available at your own risk. You should be vaccinated against "2 for the price of 1 sales" and Christmas commercials, three shots are necessary, required, compulsory, and an emigrant law to protect one from "T-Vucolosis."

(Mavis revealed her personal evaluation of the voyage on the *Hope* in a letter written on November 3, 1961 to one of the supporters of Project Hope:)

The year's experience was dynamically convincing that the "American individual" *is* one of the most effective "tools" with which to demonstrate goodwill, democracy, and America. You become crew members of a vessel whose cargo is compassion, talents of healing, and the ordinary American citizen.

My early training from life on the farm came in handy for such tricks as small containers of water under the legs of cabinets to keep the ants out of sterile supplies. We worked very hard sometimes—but then what better way is there to get to know people than to work beside them? This bears out the founding principles of HOPE.

Yes, *S.S. Hope* will sail again. All the medical staff serving on the first voyage have been requested to sail with the ship again. It is with some regret that I must admit I shall not be among the repeaters. The conditions under which I requested a year's leave to sail on the first voyage do not permit me to do so at this time.

As spokesman for the organization as a whole, let me say that your interest is greatly appreciated. In my opinion, your support is well placed when you back the People-to-People Health Foundation as a demonstration of a democratic people's compassion, and a builder of goodwill between the peoples of two nations.

(Project Hope received acclaim from former President Dwight D. Eisenhower. President John F. Kennedy renewed the Project for a second voyage. Regrettably, the trauma of the Viet Nam war soon replaced its impact. But the experience aboard the *Hope* left Mavis a changed person. Life in the U.S.A. lost its luster for her.)

4

Restlessness

Life in the comfortable, antiseptic routine of a stateside hospital didn't excite Mavis. She found her mind slipping back with nostalgia for the hectic, adventurous life aboard the *Hope*. She couldn't erase flashbacks of exotic places and faces of people who had captured more of her heart than she suspected. She also wondered what the future might hold for her and Chuck.

For months, Mavis rode the wave of adulation and acclaim that came to her after the trip to Southeast Asia. The voyage received widespread press coverage and was featured on an NBC-TV documentary, "The Good Ship Hope," on November 28, 1961. The People to People Health Foundation reported on November 29 that the *Hope* story "now fills ten books." Mavis's picture appeared in numerous publications of the voyage. Dr. Walsh, the director, made numerous references to Mavis in his book on the ship's journey.[1]

Clubs and churches invited her to speak about her experiences. Being called upon to relate her adventures acted as a further catalyst to the process that was simmering in her heart. The requests for speaking made it necessary to contact the Foreign Mission Board of the Southern Baptist Convention for materials needed for her engagements, as she related in a letter dated October 23, 1961:

On-the-spot observation of the Foreign Mission work of our church constituted some of the high points of the year's experience. Outstanding among these opportunities was the trip to the Rumah Sakit Baptis of Kederi, Indonesia. I was one of a team, two nurses and two doctors, from *Hope*, who visited and worked with Dr. Kathleen Jones and her associates when the ship was docked in Surabaja.

Dr. Jones, her staff and their work there were truly impressive and inspiring. These servants of God had won the admiration and respect, in both personal and professional aspects of the Hope Team within the hour of our arrival in Kediri.

As one might anticipate, upon arrival home there are many requests to share highlights of the voyage with various groups, particularly church groups. Some material was gathered in preparation for this; however, some poor photography on my part leaves me with inadequate coverage on many things. Herein lies the reason for contacting the Foreign Mission Board at this time.

Is my information correct? Do you have 35-mm slides available through the Board? If so, please advise me as to the most rapid method of obtaining copies.

It would be preferable to have several slides for complete coverage of the Kediri Hospital, i.e. the hospital, mission personnel, and some of their work as patients, converts, etc. In addition, I would like two or three slides of several of the other missions in Indonesia and South Vietnam, if they are available.

Thank you in advance for consideration of this request.

Sincerely,
Mavis O. Pate, R.N.
Operating Room Supervisor
Medical Center Hospital
P. O. Box 3277
Tyler, Texas

Genie, her stepsister, quickly noted Mavis's unsettled state of mind after returning from overseas. "She returned from that year quite dissatisfied with her life, though challenging and productive, even momentarily rewarding as it was. She began seeking the Lord's will in her life and during those uncertain months often would come and stay with us two or three days at a time. Van and I both worked, so we'd leave her with time alone—just rest and contemplation, with long evenings of conversation."[2]

The situation Mavis found on returning to work in Tyler threw her into a state of restlessness. The nurse who replaced her for a year did not find it easy to step aside when Mavis returned. That, coupled with the uncertainty about the future of her relationship with Chuck, led to what she termed "to concomitant personal crises, through which God worked, in spite of my obstinance, to bring me to total surrender." There followed a period of "incompleteness, marking time, waiting for what I knew not."[3]

Materialism of life in the United States, compared to the needs overseas, caused her discomfort, as she later related:

Adjustment back into the routine of the hospital and Tyler was much more difficult than I had anticipated. Doubtless it was my own restlessness and recent experiences that made me impatient with what seemed to be a narrow and materialistic view around me.[4]

Mavis did not react passively. Seeing so much need overseas and the abundance at home led her to reevaluate the use of material possessions. As a result she made a decisive decision. "For the first time I tithed all my material possessions."[5]

During a holiday visit to her sister Gwen at the homeplace in Ringgold, Mavis confided what was causing the dissatisfaction. Mavis said, "I want to be a missionary." She asked Gwen what she thought.

Gwen replied, "It's your life, and you must do what you feel is right."

"But," responded Mavis, "when I tell Mother she's going to have a fit!"

Gwen said, "That is part of it. If you want it badly enough you will do it."[6]

Mattie Oden was not unaware of the inner turmoil her daughter suffered. When discouraged, Mavis spent time with her mother, sometimes crying, sometimes sharing. At other times, she slipped out to her "secret place" to be alone with the Lord. Mattie later reflected that Mavis "left her heart over there." She dared not discourage her daughter from following God's will. But finding that will didn't come easily for "Ankle Bill."

A thyroidectomy operation in 1962 complicated Mavis's difficult readjustment to hospital work in Tyler. Then Chuck visited. Though Mavis appreciated his kindness, it became obvious to her that their future would not lead to marriage. Chuck was a seaman; he planned to sail on the second voyage of the *Hope*. He was also a Roman Catholic. His friendship meant much to Mavis, but she didn't feel that certainty needed for a permanent relationship.

Temporary comfort came as she received recognition for her professional competence and medical writing skill. She developed an operating room "prep" manual that became a standard in the field of nursing. Edward Weck & Company purchased the copyright from her in March 1963 for $500.[7] But acclaim couldn't satisfy the longing of her heart to know God's will.

Summer of 1963 arrived. The inner dissatisfaction and unrest built to the point that she knew what she must do. But as she related later, "Self was a tenacious obstacle for me!" Reading the writings of Howard Butt, Baptist layman and popular speaker, challenged her to put her faith into action. Once again she sought the counsel of her pastor, Dr. Shamburger.

As her pastor and friend, I listened to her dreams, prayed with her concerning them, planned with her to attain fulfillment in the best and fullest way. While on the *Ship Hope*, she began to weigh the needs of the world. Frustrations confronted her as she sought to find and fill the spots in the world where the need was so great.

With a combination of relief and apprehension she resigned her position at the Medical Center Hospital in Tyler. This left her with no regular income but free to pursue the impulse of her heart.

Glorieta

High in the mountains of New Mexico, overlooking Santa Fe, nestles the imposing Southern Baptist Conference Center "Glorieta." Mavis, along with Mattie, Genie, and her daughter Karen, drove the long, hot trip from Louisiana to attend Foreign Missions Week in August. The thin mountain air was exhilarating to Mavis as she talked with furloughing missionaries and Foreign Mission Board staff personnel about the possibilities of overseas service. She spent long hours discussing the pros and cons with Edna Frances Dawkins, personnel consultant for medical candidates. Edna Frances, or "Efee" as her friends called her, understood Mavis's struggle.

Sitting on a rock overlooking the lake reflecting the chapel at Glorieta, Mavis talked often with Efee about the possibility of serving one year overseas as a missionary nurse. Efee was aware of the tough mentality Mavis had developed as an operating-room nurse. They agreed to pray together and seek the Lord's leadership. Later in the week, Baker James Cauthen, executive secretary of the Foreign Mission Board, made an impassioned plea for foreign-mission service volunteers. Mavis walked forward during the final invitation hymn and presented herself for missionary service. This sealed the outward decision, but the inner struggle continued.

Now, with her mission commitment public, Mavis took steps to meet the maximum age requirement for missionary appointment. She needed to receive a year's seminary training and be appointed before her fortieth birthday. She was a bit unhappy that the Foreign Mission Board required her, a skilled medical person, top have a year of seminary studies before serving overseas. But it soon proved one of her most valuable experiences. It satisfied, as she put it, the "gnajwing, impatient, restless hunger for evicences and knowledge of God that I could not seem to lay hold of."[8]

Southwestern Baptist Theological Seminary ;is the largest of the Southern Baptist Convention graduate schools for the training of pastors, church workers, and mission candidates. Mavis moved her trailer to Forth Worth, Texas, that September of 1963 and started classes immediately. She felt, as she described it, "a peace brought by the Holy Spirit" because of her decision. She found the opportunity to study the Bible in depth and to reflect on what God was doing in her life. While writing a thesis on "the reality of God," she encountered her profoundest challenge.

The Stumbling-block Test

Southern Baptists place challenging requirements on prospective missionaries. Coupled with education and health requirements, and evidence of a clear calling to mission service, is a code of personal conduct. All of these qualifications must be verified by numerous interviews and fecommendations of people who know the candidate. Mavis could forego the occasional beer or cocktail to which she had accustomed herself in her former years. *If this is a stumbling block to others I am willing and able to let this go for the sake of the Kingdom of God,* she thought. But the habit of smoking clung to her. She had learned to smoke while a student nurse. Even though, as she put it, "I had climbed to the upper rungs of the ladder of success in my profession, I was unable to pass this 'stumbling-block test.' "9 She needed help, especially as she struggled to write her life history for the Board. *Perhaps I should confide in Edna Frances about my state of helplessness,* she thought. *If anyone would understand, it would be Efee.*

Edna Frances flew to Fort Worth for interviews with other missionary candidates. Mavis met her at the airport. On the way into the city, Mavis confided, "I can't go on with missionary appointment."

Efee replied, "Because of your smoking?"

"How did you know?" asked Mavis in surprise!

"Oh, a lot of people know you smoke," answered Efee. She didn't tell Mavis that missionaries in Southeast Asia expressed concern that Mavis's personal habits would be a "stumbling block" to the national Christians should she return as a missionary. So she explained to Mavis, "Many operating room nurses smoke, but it will be very difficult for a missionary to smoke in a Muslim culture where you may be serving." Efee made a covenant with Mavis to pray for her any time, night or day, when Mavis felt she couldn't hold out without a cigarette. She didn't realize how seriously Mavis took this offer!

The pressure to complete the life history for the Foreign Mission Board application and the term papers at seminary increased. Mavis couldn't endure without a cigarette! Once she called Efee at 1 A.M., another time at 3 A.M. for encouragement. "I just can't hold out," she gasped, and Efee prayed for her. God in His wisdom used this struggle to prove His reality to Mavis.

While she prepared the final thesis in theology for her year's study, she won the victory. In her paper, she answered the question, "How do I know that God is alive and real today?" by exclaiming, "He helped me quit smoking!" He helped her pass the "stumbling-block test." The ordeal settled her commitment to God and the calling to missions. She received new insights into herself and her mission in life, as she related in her application to the foreign Mission Board;

My ultimate goal is to achieve that which Mary Welch describes so beautifully, "the capacity always to give to others what they need to receive and to receive of others what they need to give according to the will of God."

Mavis made the following self-evaluation of her religious maturity as a result of kicking a habit through God's grace.

I am aware that I have a tendency to utilize a degree of aggressiveness to "cover-up" for any feeling of inadequacy, thus I distort what in some instances should be humbleness. I evaluate myself as a religious adolescent. I was the religious hypo-thyroid dwarf . . . convicted with the diagnosis of lack of growth for which "total-surrender pills" were prescribed.[10]

Appointment

Mavis applied for missionary service by filling in a Preliminary Information Form on February 28, 1964. She indicated that her decision resulted from an "inner unrest and conviction, evidently the work of the Holy Spirit." She listed Southeast Asia as her first choice for placement. As second choice she listed the Near East, with the possibility of Gaza. She submitted a Personal Information Form on May 4, 1964, which gave evidence of her spiritual growth and the positive effect of seminary studies:[11]

Personal Habit of Prayer

I pray each evening. Prayer is a spontaneous part of each day's activities . . . particularly in the past twelve months as through my study at seminary a new thought or aspect is clarified before me; and I feel compelled to ask forgiveness for past omissions.

Her formal application for missionary service (May 5, 1964) gave further evidence of a growing spiritual maturity as she shared her views on various aspects of the Christian life:

The Message—My concept of God—for me this is the "innate thirst for God."

What Jesus Means to Me—Depicting God's pure love and mercy will ever compound my realization of unworthiness . . . He is the majesty and power of God, the Savior. To me Jesus is God in reachable form, a Companion, one of us, ever present, yet holy and separated from us.

The Place of Prayer—A fundamental part of my communion with God. I give it most imperfect expression. Self and self-will still give me difficulty in approaching God in the right attitude, since the Spirit will not lead me to trust God for something not in His will. I find my personal desires are persistent and failure can usually be traced to my attitude in the petitions. I never cease to be awed by the power of prayer when it is in God's will.

The Church—All the redeemed elect that have been or shall be on earth and in heaven: one Body, whose head is Christ. This does not mean only the saved persons in one denomination.

Faith—A personal matter but never a private matter. Christ's reconciliation reestablishes our filial relationship to God and our fraternal relationship to one another.

Christian Responsibility to Individuals and Society—to live the new life in Christ as a continual incarnate witness to His saving grace.

The Foreign Mission Board accepted Mavis's application and recommended her for appointment to East Pakistan in July 1964. The Baptist mission there hoped to open a new hospital and wanted Mavis to assist in initiating it. Mattie, Genie, and Karen, Genie's daughter, accompanied Mavis to Richmond, Virginia for the appointment service. Following this, Mavis attended the orientation conference for new missionaries at the University of Richmond. Her spirits soared. Her decision to follow God's will began to bear fruit. But the period of testing never seemed to be over.

Waiting

Then began months of waiting for a visa to enter East Pakistan. She had planned to sail on the *S.S. President Roosevelt* on September 24,

1964, but no visa came. From time to time missionaries experienced delays in receiving visas to this Muslim country. The experience of waiting frustrated Mavis. She had to live at home with no job. She spent the time purchasing supplies for a four-year term of service in East Pakistan. She sold her furniture and trailer, and she waited. Christmas arrived—still no visa. Her spirits were low. She wanted to give gifts to friends, but lacked funds. Genie suggested that she purchase the "makings" for Christmas fruit cookies which Mavis could bake and deliver. It turned out to be a three-day project. Mavis's efficiency worked against her speed as a cook! Each package of cookies had to be artistically packed, usually with her hand-drawn or hand-cut decoration for the top. Mavis once reflected about herself: "By nature and by training, I am impatient with inefficiency."[12]

It became apparent that things might not work out for a visa to East Pakistan. Mavis expressed her willingness to serve in any other country where a nurse may be needed. As a result, Dr. Winston Crawley, Area Secretary for the Orient, Foreign Mission Board, suggested that she work in the hospital at Bangkla, Thailand, until a visa could be granted from Pakistan. The hospital expressed delight with the possibility and wrote to Dr. Crawley on January 11, 1965:

We in Bangkla believe she could make a real contribution to our hospital. We are shorthanded in nurses and Rosemary does not have enough time to adequately supervise the surgery and central supply. Therefore, Mavis could even in a short time make our surgery more efficient and less expensive. Also, she would observe a small hospital in the throes of birth and help her in avoiding some of our errors. We feel if she spent an interim period here, it would benefit the hospital here and in Pakistan both.

Mavis was overjoyed with this new opportunity, even if only for the interim. Quickly, she made plans with "Cotton" Wright, business manager at the Foreign Mission Board, to book a flight to Thailand. She said "good-bye" to the family at the Monroe, Louisiana, airport (January 31, 1965). On February 2, she found herself on Japan Air Lines flight 803 to Honolulu.

Relaxing in her seat, she wondered, *How long will this term last?*

5

East Pakistan: Part I

Interim Assignment—Bangkla, Thailand

After stopovers in Honolulu and Tokyo, Mavis arrived in Hong Kong where she received a warm welcome. Tommy Adkins, administrator of the Wallace Memorial Hospital, met her at the airport, and Mavis enjoyed renewing acquaintances with the hospital staff. "They made me feel so wanted and needed in the hospital here—ole vanity—but a part was the return to familiar places," she reflected in a letter home.[1] A chance meeting with Dr. Winston Crawley further assured her that the visa for East Pakistan would soon be granted. After a brief shopping spree she flew on to Bangkok, Thailand.

Earl Goatcher, hospital administrator, and Vera Gardner, nurse from Bangkla, met her in Bangkok. Later in Bangkla she met others of the Baptist Mission staff, Ronald Hill and family, nurse Rosemary Spessard, Dr. Orby Butcher and family, Dr. Joann Goatcher, and Dr. and Mrs. Fred Medcalf. All had children except the "three old maids," as Mavis called herself and the other nurses.

Frustration immediately set in as Mavis found herself unable to communicate in the Thai language. She admired Vera and others who had struggled with the language. "There is nothing quite as humbling as to realize that you can't communicate as you want. I just pray that God will give me the patience and ability to talk that Bengali" (the language of East Pakistan).[2]

Thai customs made her nostalgic for childhood days, especially removing one's shoes at the door and going barefoot in the house. She learned the taboos, those gestures considered impolite and offensive, such as pointing with the foot and standing with hands on one's hips. She experienced the frustration of needing four signatures for a driver's license and the fact that in Thailand you do not question an official, even if you want to uphold a principle.[3]

Mavis found Thai food delicious and interesting. She enjoyed "san-ke-ahh," a custard made in a green coconut shell with the milk of the coconut. Also green mango pie—very much like green apple pie, and ripe mango ice cream. A mouth-watering main dish of "wee-thio"—broad, one-inch noodles with cabbage, shrimp, pork and beef, pepper and vinegar, and "nain blah" fish sauce reminded her of Louisiana delicacies. Another was "cow pok," fried rice with onions and meat in a pan, sauteed.

Mavis learned that the Thai people celebrate life and death differently than in the West. She attended a wedding in which the couple stood for the reception and well-wishers poured water over the couple's hands as they passed by. Then she witnessed a Buddhist funeral. They cleaned the body, then wrapped and placed it in a coffin on an altar in the home. The Buddhist monk indicated the proper time to remove the flesh and cremate the bones.

En route to work, Mavis often passed a young goat herder with a transistor radio, a graphic example of the old and new in the Orient. She assisted Orby Butcher and Rosemary Spessard with surgery, reorganized the operating room and OB department, and trained the Thai nurses in operating room procedures. Occasionally life in Bangkla reminded her of life aboard the *S.S. Hope.* It required extra patience—especially when she discovered that bees had swarmed and were making a hive in the sterilizing room! After a busy day she remarked, "Wow, I'm worn out! Can I really be a missionary nurse?—only by God's grace and love—not mine![4]

She finally received word that her visa to East Pakistan had been authorized. Mavis found it particularly hard to wait for news and instructions. "There are three things I can't quite get used to in this work:

(1) Everyone knows your news before you do.
(2) No one gives direct, specific answers to questions for one of two

reasons—the situation may change within the next few hours, or they do not wish to appear aggressive.

(3) The dogs in the neighborhood howl every once in a while as though they are being dreadfully mistreated."[5]

Sunday, March 14, 1965, marked a banner day in the life of the Thailand Baptist Mission. Over 100 people from around the country gathered at the bridge near Bangkla for a baptismal service. Mavis noted that the leader delayed the service until all could arrive, some even coming on bicycles. Seven new believers proclaimed their faith by baptism, and the Bangkla Baptist Church was constituted *underneath* the Goatcher's home built on stilts, typical of Thai homes.[6]

A trip into Bangkok with the Butchers offered Mavis her first experience in driving in Thailand. "Driving in that place! On the wrong side of the street! No traffic lights! No lanes! And me not knowing the city!" She spared herself the agony when the Butcher's Cortina broke down. All three adults and three children piled into Rosemary Spessard's Volkswagen "beetle." The trip that ordinarily took an hour and a half took them four hours! Mavis mused, "They keep telling me you have to 'play it by ear' (better laid plans of mice and men go astray) *but* my theory is that you never know what goal you have missed if you don't set one up to shoot at! I do have moments that remind me of the frustrations on board that ship called *Hope*—more patience I need."[7]

As she prepared to leave for East Pakistan, there was a special meeting to bid farewell to Ronald and Evelyn Hill who were leaving for their furlough. To her surprise the mission included Mavis in the farewell and gave her a lovely ruby princess ring as a gift. To her delight, the Thai nurses she had trained during her short stay showed up, along with Rosemary, to see her off. March 22, 1965 and it was on to East Pakistan!

Dacca—Orientation

Greeting a new missionary is always a grand event for a small mission in a Muslim country. Trueman Moore, Baptist missionary, helped Mavis through customs at the airport. Then the surprise—the entire East Pakistan Baptist Mission gathered to meet her! The Rythers,

Teels, Moores, Carneys, Johnsons, Becketts, and Ruth Dickerson immediately adopted Mavis into "the family."

The next day the missionary families gathered for a covered dish supper in Mavis's honor. Charles Beckett presented a devotion after dinner and told her that one of the MKs (missionary kids) prayed last week "that Aunt Mavis may receive her visa." A rainstorm in the midst of the celebration didn't dampen their spirits.

Orientation began in earnest. *No hurry, but here's your hat, there's the door,* thought Mavis as Charles Beckett explained all that would be expected of her. "Don't rush into language school but meet your language teachers, get your books, read the minutes of the Mission from its beginning, and visit all Baptist work in East Pakistan in the next two months." So she visited the mission office, met her language teachers, picked up a brief outline of language school, received expense account forms from the treasurer, attended a prayer meeting, and heard a lecture on Islam—*all in one day!*

Orientation and language study receive priority in Southern Baptist missions. Experience proves that a person's adaptability and effectiveness in a foreign culture depend on : (1) acquiring an adequate grasp of the new culture and (2) its language. Preparation makes life overseas far more fulfilling. Mavis determined to make the best of it. Reading the mission minutes bored her, but attending a Pakistani wedding party made up for it!

On the plane to Dacca, Mavis met a stately Pakistani lady, Mrs. Sheik, who invited her to her son's wedding. The festivities began with a party at her daughter's home. Mavis was surprised it was an informal come-and-go affair. She soon learned why. The son provides the clothes and jewelry for his bride-to-be. The eight different "saris" (wraparound dresses) and gold costume jewelry are laid out for all to see. Four hired women provided the music. After an hour of chit-chat, everyone participates in an unusual tradition. There are six or eight buckets of water in the yard, each with a different color of food dye in it. With a little frolic and horseplay, the women and children start pouring the water on each other! Then they invited Mavis outside, and graciously explained, "You will probably want to watch." In a while when many were drenched and looking like Easter eggs, they came inside to change clothes! Refreshments of American soft drinks were offered, but the specialty is milk with coloring added, with a bit of fruit mixed in for flavor. Milk was scarce and expensive and drunk only by the elite.[8]

The crush of humanity and the male-dominated society surprised Mavis as she went to the market in old Dacca. "No words will describe it—people, people, people. It is utter calamity. What do they have to live for?" She found that women hesitate to visit the market because they are treated badly and called ugly names. So the women usually waited until the afternoon, after the male cooks had bought the best portions of meat. The women were in "purdah" (wearing the veil). Most of the progressive younger generation did not, but occasionally out of respect and veneration for their families some young women wear the veil. Mavis heard men explain, "Wife kept in 'purdah' until parents pass away out of respect for them!"[9]

(This was a quarter of a century ago, and customs have changed, but many vestiges remain in Muslim countries.) In contrast, she was surprised to discover the characteristics of men in a society that subjugates women. Mavis observed the men walking down the street holding hands with each other. Some painted their fingernails and let the little fingernail grow long in order to hook with the fingernail of their friends. Chivalry was shown toward other men rather than toward women as in Western society.[10]

The shocking realization of the resistance of the Muslim culture to the Gospel became even more apparent when a missionary friend related the story of Khadija, a Muslim girl who visited a Christian dispensary not far from her village:

"Khadija heard the Bible women tell about Jesus. She argued but agreed to take a Bible and study it. The missionary agreed to read her Quran (Koran) and to be open to follow the one that led to the truth. After a year's study she remarked, "Both of these great religions cannot be true. I will continue to search until I am convinced of one or the other, and then I will live by that one." Then one day she appeared with the dawn of truth lighting her face. The Bible held the truth! She believed Jesus Christ was her Savior, and she wanted to make a profession of faith and be baptized! But the matter of her family and her children had to be faced. If she were to declare her faith openly, her children would be taken from her and she might face threat of death. With these realities facing her she returned to her village. A few months later, two of Khadija's fellow Christians visited her sister's home. They were startled when at sight of them sobs burst forth from the woman. It appeared that Khadija had never hidden her faith from her relatives. She had been put out of her home and had her property confiscated. They had locked her in a room, but she persisted in reading the Bible so loudly that passersby could hear. She was finally silenced, probably by poisoning. The sister learned of her death two days after the burial.

"This tragic, but oft-repeated, tale of persecution of converts in a Muslim land reminded Mavis of the high price paid by those who dare to profess Christ in that culture. The official government policy varies, of course, from country to country. The opposition became personal when Mavis learned about the difficulties the Mission was facing trying to gain permission to build the new hospital. She encouraged herself with the prayer, "May God grant me patience and wisdom at this time, here in this place, for whatever is His purpose, even if it is without visible results at the moment."[11]

Eid Al-Adha, Muslim Feast

The panorama in front of Mavis's window in April 1965 was unbelievable! It was the preparation day for the "Eid," a Muslim holiday. Cows, bullocks, goats, and other animals with decorated bridles paraded by to the stadium. One man was leading a pink goat! The Muslim high holiday of "Eid Al-Adha" (pronounced "azha") or the Feast of the Sacrifice of Abraham was being observed. Muslims believe that Abraham started to sacrifice Ishmael and not Isaac.

Jeanne Beckett, missionary doctor, escorted Mavis to her first day of language school and introduced her to the teachers. She was to learn basic Bengali from Simon Sircar, vocabulary through pictures with Miss Renu Sircar, and conversation from Banerjee. The next day Charles Beckett drove her downtown for the "Eid."

Everyone greets his friends with "Eid Mubarak," translated "Have a happy and successful festival!" Prayers had already begun at 7:30

A.M. in the mosques and the outer stadium. The long lines of men kneeling side by side with their foreheads touching the ground, facing toward Mecca, impressed Mavis. There is a unity in the rituals of Islam. After the prayers a sermon is delivered. Beggars line the entrance to the mosques anticipating generous offerings on this feast day, since Muslims are admonished to help the poor.[12]

The next day was another holiday, the celebration of the Muslim New Year of 1372. Muslims traditionally date their calendar from the year of the "Hijrah" (Hejirah) or the escape of the prophet Muhammed from Mecca to Medina in the year 622 A.D. Pakistani businessmen celebrate the tradition of "hal khata," by opening new account books and offering sweets to clients.

Most missionaries in a foreign culture suffer "culture shock" or a degree of depression, loneliness, and general "let down." It sneaks in at different times for different people, but it invariably comes. For Mavis, perhaps it was brought on by the pain of an abscessed tooth, or the wind and rain of the seasonal winds. She recorded in her diary on May 6, 1965: "Another trip to the market for the week's supplies. Cultural shock was evident in impatience and persecution complex." She began to feel the gnawing ache of separation from home. Her baggage hadn't arrived, and her depression was not unwarranted as can be seen by the red-tape she endured to retrieve it.

1. Trip almost to airport—back to house to get declaration slip.
2. Trip to airport—assured we must go to downtown office to get original of shipping paper.
3. Trip downtown—paper not there. Call to airport finds paper on desk there.
4. Trip back to airport—Get paper, bags, and boy to accompany us to freight and customs office.
5. Trip to air freight—from 12:30 to 2:30 we are assured we will not be able to get shipment today. We urge them to try. They continue as usual or at slower pace. Agents fill out paper (five copies—no carbon used), many arguments to prevent claiming all personal-effects allowance of $200, then none left for sea freight. His superior checks, sends

to customs officer . . . he checks, same argument about amount. District customs officer checks, then back to customs office to inspect bags, then back to district officer who checks passes—then says, "You will not be able to get these today. You must go to airport, get superintendent of customs to sign, go to Central Security to get assistant customs collector to sign, and then come back here. Asked if superintendent's office is open, says yes.
6. Trip to airport—to find superintendent gone for the day, and his assistant cannot sign.

Little wonder that next day Mavis woke with a high fever and what she claims was "culture shock and withdrawal symptoms." She couldn't face church and Sunday School in Bengali. Instead she went to the evening services in English. Finally she checked out her baggage with only three more trips and the usual delays!

A terrific storm blew up the next evening. Trees came crashing down, shutters and gates tore off, and half the brick walls in town were destroyed. Many of the missionary homes suffered flooding. The homes of poorer Pakistanis suffered more devastation, and many could be seen propping up their thatched roofs. Mavis marveled that it did not deter the holiday parades. People celebrated the martyrdom of Ali and Hussein, prophets. Young boys with sticks fought mock sword fights in the streets in memory of the ancient Battle of Karbala. *How will I ever understand these people, or get them to understand me?* she asked herself.

Bengali Language Study

Despite the unsettling effect of adapting to the new culture, Mavis gave her best—reluctantly—to study Bengali. It was not easy for her or for the teacher. Her inquisitive and precise mind did not yield easily to generalizations, of which the Oriental world is full. She always wanted to know the reason for things. Her mind-set called for an explanation! Thomas and Gloria Thurman studied with her and remembered her always wanting to know "why" certain words and phrases were spoken in a certain way. One teacher didn't know the "why" of many grammar rules. Mavis commented, "But there *has* to be a reason why!" The teacher replied, "If just sounds sweet to our ears." That didn't satisfy Mavis. She sat with her arms folded, staring straight at the teacher until it was clear he couldn't answer. Then she rushed out of the room! The teacher collected himself for ten minutes before going to the next class!

Language study was so intensive and confining Mavis had to hire a maid and a cook. She and the local Pakistanis had their differences. She hired a cook who refused to shop in the market. One day Mavis went to the market alone and bought two live chickens just to prove she could do it. They were hardly big enough for the broiler. She wrote, "I felt so sorry for them I would have turned them loose when I got home if I had not spent all my money."[14] To make matters worse, after a tongue-twisting day in language study she came home to find the chickens not cleaned properly and blood all over the kitchen floor. She decided then that she needed a cook who would do the marketing and clean up after himself. One cook after another quit and dutifully sent a friend to fill in as long as they both could stand it!

A much-needed mission retreat interrupted language study. By this time Mavis had gained notoriety for her food preservation techniques which she transferred from Louisiana to Pakistan. She left "twenty-one-day pickles" in a churn to cure during the mission retreat. Upon returning she started to prepare her jars for the pickles. Oh, oh. The day after she left for the meeting, the helper noticed foam on the pickles, so she carefully washed the pickles every day! Mavis sat quietly for a while, put up her jars, and threw the pickles out. She was later heard mumbling, "The only certainty is the uncertainty of it all!"

Christmas in August

Despite the cultural adjustments and frustrations in Pakistan, as well as a tendency to procrastinate, Mavis made a 93 on her language exam. As with other missionaries, language study is a long-term process, often interrupted by the unexpected. "Christmas in August" is one of those welcome interruptions. Mavis's shipment of furniture and supplies finally arrived. "I'm sitting in my very own orange chair, and I slept *beside* my beautiful blue bed (I didn't sleep on it because I was too tired to put on the linen last night, and it's almost too pretty to sleep on)." The touch of the familiar gave her pangs of homesickness. As she related to a sick relative, "At a time like this the slowness of communication is so exasperating. I would love to be able to pick up the phone and talk with you."[15]

The annual mission meeting is another necessary interruption. Southern Baptists operate their missions uniquely, characteristics of their democratic life-style. Each mission in a foreign country exercises a high degree of autonomy. The Foreign Mission Board depends on the missionaries in a particular country to plan strategy, place personnel, elect officers, and determine budgets in keeping with the particular needs of that country. They do this officially at an annual meeting. All missionaries in the country are required to attend. They usually enjoy it, despite the hours of preparation for reports. It is a time of fellowship and spiritual nourishment, in addition to decision-making.

Mavis learned at her first annual meeting that missionaries meet and differ like other people! After a tedious, heated session she said, "The only reason we make plans is to have something to change!" As a result of that meeting the mission elected Mavis as hospitality chairman of the Dacca station, which later developed into a full-time job when the mission established a guest house.

Back into language study, Mavis began to feel the drag of keeping up. She even experimented with playing Bengali tapes while she slept, but with no audible results!

An unexpected gift lifted her spirits. Phil Parshall, Baptist missionary of another mission, left behind a five-year-old female dachshund who needed to find a home. This new companion delighted Mavis. It reminded her of "Duke" from years ago, affectionate, intelligent, and almost human. Somehow she later obtained another dachshund. The MKs loved to visit her and enjoyed her treats and dachshunds—perhaps because the dogs loved peanut brittle and bananas as much as they did.

Evacuation—Manila, Philippines

An unexpected turn of events on the borders of Pakistan interrupted language study. The formation of the state of Pakistan by partition (August 1947) had strained relations with India. Eighteen years later unrest erupted into open war. India bombed Dacca and other Pakistani cities. The Baptist mission curtailed work due to blackout and curfew conditions. The American Consulate notified the mission on September 8, 1965, that all non-essential personnel were advised to evacuate to Manila, Philippines, because of the hostilities. The Executive Committee of the Baptist Mission met and voted for all the women and children to evacuate and for Dr. J. W. "Dub" Carney to accompany them. The other men elected to stay and watch the situation and follow later if necessary. The local Pakistanis were surprised that all did not leave.

As the plane took off for Manila (September 19, 1965) Mavis was more concerned about what the folks back home were thinking than about her own safety!

Phil Anderson, music missionary, met the plane at the Manila airport and assisted the group in processing for their temporary stay. Mary Lucille Saunders welcomed Mavis and gave her the full run of the house, making her feel at home. She even planned meals to include green vegetables, fruit, bacon, bologna, salami, and cereals— items not available in Pakistan. A visit to the Baptist Bookstore found the staff friendly and helpful. After settling in, the "Pakistan Mission in Exile" issued a news release to assure all the folks back home that they were safe.

It was refreshing to see the country, to fellowship with the Philippine missionaries, and to visit in their churches. A trip to volcanic Lake Taal and the scenic mountain town of Baguio impressed Mavis. The scenery there and fellowship with missionary friends reminded her of Glorieta, New Mexico. Being out of Pakistan renewed her spirits. She related to the family back home:

Overall, the country impresses me as being about 25 years ahead of Pakistan in social, cultural, and industrial progress. The people you see as you walk down the street, or pass them on the road, or wherever, have a much happier countenance. And there is much more evidence of their happiness and gaiety in the beauty of their countryside, the lovely colors every place, and the different types of art.

The Philippine mission planned a special trip to Mati for Dr. "Dub"

Carney and Mavis to visit the Baptist Hospital and to be of assistance while they were in the country. But before this trip could be finalized Mavis received a telegram from Earl Goatcher in Thailand, saying, "We have requested Dr. Crawley to let you stay in Bangkla temporarily if satisfactory with you."

It thrilled her to feel wanted and useful again. She and "Dub" traveled to Mati and spent several days assisting in the hospital and sharing inspiration in the morning devotion times. In a special meeting with Dr. Crawley (October 26, 1965) they decided for "Dub" to remain in Mati and for Mavis to go on to Bangkla until the situation in Pakistan stabilized. Dr. Crawley emphasized the Foreign Mission Board policy in such situations: "not to close doors but if doors closed to accept and move on to something else." So, once again, Mavis found one door temporarily closed and another opened.

Before flying to Thailand, Mavis spent a few days with the Todd Hamilton family. Todd was a dedicated church developer. Mavis, Todd and a group of students motored into Parasapas, a village that requested a preaching team to share the gospel with them. After arriving and making introductions, the group conducted a meeting on the spot. They sang for the children and preached through an interpreter. Eleven men raised their hands indicating they wanted to invite Jesus into their hearts! The students then made plans for follow-up meetings and instruction of new believers. What a marked contrast to the difficulties one faced in Pakistan![18]

Back to Bangkla

The "welcoming committee" in Bangkok surprised Mavis. Present to meet her were the Loflands, Ruth Dickerson, and Ralph Marshall from Bangkok and Vera Gardner, Dora Howard, and Nom the seamstress from the hospital in Bangkla. She spent the weekend securing an official entry visa and renewing acquaintances with the Roland Hills, Judson Lennons, and other missionary friends in Bangkok. Mavis was asking, "How much time will I be allowed in Bangkla as it seems that return to East Pakistan might be near?" But a cloud of doubt still loomed over the future of hospital work in East Pakistan. Early in her career Mavis was becoming an itinerant missionary.

Arriving at the hospital in Bangkla, Mavis received an even more enthusiastic welcome. Shortly she found herself involved in "scrubbing" for a caesarean section. The following days she performed such chores as to trim the ear of a leprosy patient, set up for a lacerated leg, and explore a knee for a bullet. The hospital staff was concerned about having too many superficial infections. Mavis attempted to help improve sterilization techniques. One of the hangups in medical missions is having so much to do and so little time to do it! When nurses are not available the doctors have to do the work, and vice versa. Fortunately, Mavis knew how to use her talents even over a short term. She was so busy tidying up around the hospital she completely forgot when Thanksgiving rolled around.

Return to Pakistan

The all clear for return to Pakistan came on December 1, 1965. Pakistani leader Ayub Khan expected to visit the U.S. soon to confer with President Lyndon Johnson. Government employees were returning to work. Rationing of gas and food was no longer necessary, but there was some shortage of rice. The government prohibited trips to border areas and clamped down on aggressive evangelism, though it allowed church meetings. The hospital had not yet received approval, but the mission stayed hopeful. In its interim mission personnel thought of sponsoring a clinic to utilize medical personnel on the field. On the basis of these certainties, or uncertainties, Mavis and the other missionaries returned to Pakistan.[19]

Ecstatic faces greeted Mavis at church in Dacca on Sunday, December 5, 1965. "When you left we did not expect you ever to return to Pakistan," remarked her Pakistani friends. The atmosphere in the country was decidedly anti-American. She had discerned an anti-American and anti-missionary slant in the local press before leaving. Then the country openly espoused friendship with Communist China. Because missionaries worked closely with the local population, their movements were hedged in until permits could be issued for travel outside of Dacca. To the relief of the mission the permits were finally granted. Families rejoiced as they returned to their homes and renewed their work.

The arrival of Thomas and Gloria Thurman, new appointees to Pakistan, was special for Mavis. She felt a closeness to them and believed that "the enthusiasm and sincerity of the Thurmans are infectious and what the Pakistan Mission needs."[20] Perhaps the friendship came naturally because of a shared love for country ham and cornbread dressing! They managed to buy a ham from the local Hindu "bootlegger," since pork is not sold on the open market in a Muslim country.

Mavis's Bengali friends celebrated Christmas in the usual fashion at the Immanuel Baptist Church in Dacca. After a morning worship service and caroling with a sound truck, the church gathered at the Trueman Moore home for a love feast. They served Pakistani-style with everyone seated or kneeling on mats. Everyone ate rice and curry with their hands, the local custom.

Mavis had a tough time returning to language study after the Christmas holidays. Her gregarious nature attracted others to drop by, and they in turn invited her for visits. So many were visiting her that she was covered up with household chores. When the mission officially opened the guest house, it relieved some of the pressure on her. There was comfort in that the Thurmans studied language with her as "fellow sufferers." Dr. Crawley on his occasional trips listened to her complaints and tried to encourage her with such advice as, "Yes, that is why you are here, you know, because we felt that you were mature enough to face the difficulties if anyone was." More times than one the encouraging word or mild rebuke of the area director kept a first-term missionary on the field. Mavis reacted, "Now, what is a feller to do but get up Monday morning and dig in again! No complaint except I just don't wanna study Bengali. I need the pressure of having to teach OR techniques tomorrow in Bengali!"[21]

Language study did at times pay off unexpectedly. Mavis's spirits lifted when she found out what her name meant in Bengali. She wrote to her mother, "After all these years I have learned why I am called 'Bill.' I learned the other day that my name 'Mavis' in Bengali means 'Bul Bul,' a bird with a beautiful song, and we must have changed it to Bill!"[22]

The difficult adjustment didn't turn her from sensitivity to the needs around her. She heard about a new Christian whose family turned him out. He needed financial assistance to study in a technical college. She checked out the story and decided to commit half of her tithe, anonymously, to assist the young man. The plight of a young Christian wife also deeply touched her. She had committed suicide by pouring kerosene on her body and setting herself on fire. There was no opportunity to assist the poor girl. Mavis wondered what bitterness or anguish caused such a tragic act, which is unfortunately common in the East.

Hospital Shelved

Amid mounting anti-American propaganda in the news and glowing reports of aid from Red China, the East Pakistan Mission continued to pursue the permit to build the hospital. The local people appealed to the governor to allow the construction. Every appeal, no matter through what channel, ran into a dead end. The existing Catholic hospital came under pressure not to proselyte or to proclaim their religion. Finally, in April 1966, the mission received word to "let sleeping dogs lie." The obstacle was political, and no manner of appeal would receive the governor's approval. Coupled with a bad case of the "two-bucket" dysentery, Mavis was crushed. The government also denied Dora Howard's visa. Others ran into the same obstacles.

As always Mavis turned to the Lord to seek direction. Mary Welch's book *The Golden Key* meant much to her through this difficult period. The problem with language study and the "wall" she felt with the language teacher caused her to admit, "I cannot overcome it alone. Only God can. His help I seek!"[23] Naturally, she questioned her calling to missions as she found herself setting up housekeeping and then receiving the bad news about the hospital. "Whoever told me I wanted to see the world? That wasn't what God said, was it? He just said, 'go and wait,' and 'I'll let you know what to do next,' O.K., so I will!"[24] The following words sent to her loved ones at home that Easter revealed the inner desires of her heart:

> May He whose love eternal
> Is the symbol of true perfection

Fill your hearts this Easter
With the joy of the Resurrection.

—Author Unknown

Outpatient Clinic—Bogra

Missionaries are resilient. They bounce back most of the time. An invitation came for Mavis to assist in a Church of God outpatient clinic in Bogra located in the northwestern part of the country. This gave her a chance to think over the possibility of transfer to another field and to escape the subtle, but increasing, political harassment of missionaries in Dacca. The mission approved her going to Bogra from May 12 to June 21 in order to relieve Donna Sleamon who would be on vacation.

Mavis immediately began to view the results of Bengali study as she put her scant knowledge into practice. Her experience is typical of other missionaries who struggle to learn a foreign language:[25]

I am in a hospital—well, out-patient clinic mostly, but I go by the hospital daily—and it lets me feel a little necessary again. I feel like I have my feet on the ground at least until I start trying to talk to these village women about why they came to see the doctor. It is a strange thing, but the only Bengalis I feel I have any rapport with are the two and three-year-olds! We communicate pretty well! There was a day or two last week when I felt that the only accomplishment I could claim was that I had entertained the patients and the nurse attendants while Dr. Gilbert chatted along amiably and with complete ease to the steady stream of patients . . . My method has been to try to write down the pertinent questions in such a way that they can give a yes or no answer and then try to get them to understand my Bengali enough to . . . to give a yes or no answer. Sometimes that works but more often than not when they grasp that you are saying a word or two of Bengali they let loose a torrent of words, three of which I may have caught.

(Bengali study meant going to class by 6:30 A.M., but Mavis relished seeing her communications skills pay off. Since Dr. Fidelia Gilbert was the only other foreigner around, it meant spending more time

with the local workers. Mavis even ended up counting money in Bengali! She was delighted to be training the Bengali nurses. The missionaries' furloughs required the locals to handle more responsibility. Mavis felt they were equal to the task.)
The fellowship with Dr. Gilbert refreshed them. They often visited the nearby Hindu pottery-making village. The handmade pottery reminded Mavis of the illustrations of the potter's wheel in the Bible. The scenery around the hospital called to mind Rudyard Kipling's *Kim*, which she had begun reading in Bogra:[26]

It speaks of the women traveling on the road in ox carts with curtains all around so that no one sees them. That reminds me of the parking lot of the hospital . . . On a full clinic day there will be ten or twelve ox carts out under the trees with the oxen tethered out, a pallet under the cart for the children. At mealtime they build fires and cook their food.

Bogra gave Mavis the chance to sample new foods. Milk clabber called "doughy" reminded her of good tart buttermilk. "Piash," a kind of rice pudding and fried "dahl," a small bean about 1/10th the size of butterbeans are popular. Because of the lack of good beef they eat lots of fried bananas, fried eggplant, and goat, mutton, chicken, and fish. The custom is for one to invite you to "eat rice" with them rather than eat dinner. The host or hostess calls at the guest's home, and then escorts the guest to the rice snack.

The experience in Bogra helped Mavis better to understand the local culture. It enabled her to adapt somewhat to the slower pace of East Pakistan. She found herself "going native" more and more every day. Reflecting on this slow change she related:[27]

I saw an excellent statement the other day . . . "It is said that if one continually butts his head against a brick wall he eventually reaches the point where he does not charge as hard as he once did." That fits the situation, I think. I'm not charging so hard these days!

Bengali Wedding

On returning to Dacca, Mavis discovered to her glee that her language teacher canceled classes and invited her to his wedding in Faridpur! The wedding signified an important event for the East Pakistan church since he pastored the church in Dacca. Due to difficulty in arranging flights, Mavis drove down to Faridpur with Tom and Gloria Thurman.[28]

In Faridpur we received, delivered by hand, our engraved invitation to the wedding and learned that the "bathing" of the bride and groom would be sometime that morning. The "bathing" is a tradition that I find about as much basis for as our throwing rice or tying old shoes on the car. All the women of both wedding parties get together and grind the various spices of different colors, go to the local tank, get water, and proceed to douse the groom (first at his house). In the process everyone is very happy, festive, and playful. Consequently everyone gets doused! After the groom is "bathed" they proceed to do the same to the bride at her house. A specific time is set for this event . . . like 10 A.M. for the groom and it comes off about 1:30; for the bride at about 2:30 (the wedding was to be about 4:00 but was about 5:00). This is the Oriental concept of time for you! The actual service was not too different from ours in form. We sat on the floor since that is the custom in the Faridpur church (some have chairs), they used two rings, and the service concluded with the bride and groom going over to a table to sign the register rather than kissing and having the recessional down the aisle. The crowd mills around and most of them get outside the church and wait. An important tradition is for the young male members of the bride's party to close and lock the departing door. Oriental-style bargaining must go on for fifteen minutes or longer until the groom pays them off to open the door and let them leave. After the wedding the newlyweds made a trip through town, then to the bride's house for the "feeding." The bride and groom sit on the floor in wedding array. Friends come by and give them a bite of sweet and a drink of water. The guest feeds them . . . don't you know the front of the bride's wedding sari was spoiled with drippings? (This is well wishing for happiness and plenty). We went to pick them up next morning at the bride's house and take them to the groom's parent's house for the day's activities which ended with the feast that night.

(The festivities over, Mavis returned with the Thurmans to Dacca to attend the annual mission meeting. Sitting was a battle for endurance since Mavis fell down her steps, and, as she described it, suffered a "sore tail." However, it didn't prevent the mission from electing her secretary of the annual meeting!)

Holy Family Hospital

Mavis passed by the Holy Family Hospital one day and discussed with the director of nursing the possibility of working with them part-time in the OR or any way she might be needed. The director was enthusiastic. The personnel committee of the Mission gave the go-ahead and approved the suggestion (July 1966). After finishing the annual meeting minutes, she set up a schedule for language study and part-time work at the hospital.

Rapport between Catholics and Protestants improved following the liberalizing actions of the Vatican II Council. Pope John XXIII appeared to lead the church closer to the Scriptures, allowed Mass in the local languages, and generally opened the Roman Catholic Church to a new movement of the Holy Spirit. Many missionaries in the 1960s discovered a Catholic Church that in many areas was no longer hostile to Protestant missions. Catholics were more open to dialogue. Mavis had the added advantage of being a highly qualified professional nurse. This gave her added rapport with the medical staff at Holy Family Hospital.

After her discouraging experiences with household help, Mavis developed a rather negative attitude about the possibility of training the East Pakistanis in medical proficiency. Her exposure at Holy Family helped to alter her thinking . . .[29]

Back to my pleasant experience getting inside a hospital again. I was very encouraged and pleased to see, after observing the team while they were doing a removal of a gall bladder, that "these individuals" can be trained to function in what we have come to consider an acceptable way in like situations. I was really beginning to question this but of course about the only thing I had to base a view on was the household helpers and their varied abilities . . . All in all, I was encouraged by the efficiency and effectiveness I noted on the part of the girls in the OR. As the Sister said, "It took much time and patience." Maybe I'm still going to that patience school, or if not I should be.

"Patience school" at Holy Family affirmed Mavis. The atmosphere and smell of a hospital made her feel at home. The Sisters of Medical Missions of Philadelphia who operated the hospital gave her the task of identifying stock instruments. Mavis had fun because, as she related, "People are generous and give the Mission Hospital all the old junk they have around and don't know what to do with it." She enjoyed it so much that the four or five hours she spent on her workday passed by quickly.

It was not long before they asked Mavis to teach OR techniques to several nursing students at Holy Family. Despite the fact that another cook had quit, she invited four of the nursing students from the hospital to lunch. She had met two of the girls in Bogra. It turned out to be a most enlightening experience:[30]

Well, I say, it is difficult to keep up with the younger generation these days, especially when they frustrate in another language . . . I tried to entertain with "Spill and Spell" and with "Cubic" which held them for a little while. But then their curiosity got the best of them, and *I found them in my bedroom trying on things.* Loss of face or no, I had to tell them that this was not considered polite where I came from. Other than that, all went well, and I think I had enough rice to keep them from getting hungry before the evening meal.

(This would not to be the last time she caught nursing students trying on her clothes. It added to the endless variety of her Pakistani memories.)

Maneuvering in the downtown traffic of Dacca, combined with the oppressive heat, was a formidable challenge:[31]

There seems to be no time when the lights are not blinding you. Once I thought a building was on fire as pedestrians came out of the fog with kerchiefs to their noses, and I could not see past the dark cloud settling on the street. As I got closer, I realized it was only a bus starting up from the bus stop. Don't know what he was using for fuel. That couldn't be someone coming toward me on this, my side of a boulevard street. Oh yes, it is! A pedal rickshaw with no light! And there is a cow calmly lying, chewing her cud, in the street beside the middle isle. That is just part of the excitement of driving downtown on any evening.

A swell of frustrations built up inside Mavis despite the fellowship she experienced with the Sisters at Holy Family Hospital. She had been away from home for nearly two years. The constant strain of adapting to an unfamiliar culture, the demands of people who showed up at her door unexpectedly, and the preparations to accommodate missionary friends all welled up. Melancholy expressions on the people's faces in the streets troubled her spirit. When the Thurmans arrived to prepare for an anticipated trip to Nepal, the dam burst. What she called her "depression other than in the Bay of Bengal" erupted in an inexplicable crying jag. The Thurmans endured sympathetically. Mavis decided to quit language study until after taking local leave. Nepal offered the respite she needed.

Nepal—Land of the Idols

The DC-3 winged over snowcapped mountains to land in the beautiful valley of Kathmandu. Mavis, along with Dr. Fidelia Gilbert from Bogra, and the Thurmans, anticipated a change of pace in this remote country high in the Himalayas. She was amazed at the contrast between Nepal and East Pakistan:[32]

I think I have probably learned more about the Hindu and Buddhist practices than ever before on this trip. It makes one more grateful than ever to be the citizen of a Christian nation and it makes one realize the tremendous needs of this world—then the feeling so inadequate to meet any of those needs . . . Hate to leave the marvelous November-like climate and dry atmosphere. It may still be flooding in Dacca. Hate to get back where I can't even take an evening walk without stares and sneers that drive one inside the house again. Didn't realize how close we stay and how good it is to have other women folk on the streets with you . . . The mountain scenery is gorgeous, and the people are open, friendly, and receptive.

Mavis's American Indian blood attracted the Nepalese. Her high cheekbones and slanted eyes caught their attention. The local people asked her several times if she were Mexican, Vietnamese, Japanese, or Russian!)

The high altitude and change of climate affected Tom Thurman who became ill with a sore throat and fever. This gave Mavis a chance to become acquainted with the United Mission Hospital, the only Protestant mission work in Nepal. It was and is against the law to change one's religion on the national registration and unlawful to proselytize in this country.

The magnificent palaces offered endless hours of touring pleasure. Mavis marveled at how such structures could have been built with materials carried on the backs of men over the forbidding mountains and over rope bridges. But the idolatry of the people impacted her the most:[33]

At first in Nepal, the Hindu and Buddhist temples are interesting and grossly very pretty to see; but after seeing one on every street corner and several smaller ones in between; after seeing the accumulated dirt and refuse from the offering, etc., around and about them; after seeing the monkeys, goats, cows, and birds eating the offerings left there for the gods; after seeing the hideousness of most of the man-made idols and wondering at the imagination that created such a representative of their own creator, one begins to see the sameness of each and every temple, the filth they accumulate, the depressive atmosphere they engender, and it makes one glad to leave the "Land of the Idols." It appears that every facet of life is involved in making, worshiping, fearing, or offering to the idols. We should give thanks for the simplicity, the beauty, and the fresh clean, air of God's true Universal Church in the wide-open Kingdom of God.

As the plane winged back to Dacca, Mavis thought, *I wish that I had followed the advice of the Foreign Mission Board to take at least thirty days leave every year!* She did not want to return, but she did. And God would reward her in unexpected ways.

The stark paganism of Nepal stirred something deep in her spirit, even as the hot East Pakistani wind blew away the chill of the Nepal mountain air. Her devotional studies deepened:[34]

Dr. Crayford's *The Overflowing Life* and McConkey's *The Threefold Secret of the Holy Spirit* seem to have been sent to meet my need at present. We *receive* the Holy Spirit when we repent and believe on Jesus Christ, but we are *filled* with the Holy Spirit only when we surrender all self-will to God's will. I must come to the point of surrendering my possessions, my expectations, my aims, and my goals if these be not according to His will. This I have not been able to do yet.

(New insights and new ministries followed as she searched for His will for her life.)

6

East Pakistan: Part II

New Insights

Her dreaded language exam was set for October 15, 1966. But before the day arrived Mavis found herself embroiled in a church dispute involving her language teacher who was also the pastor. She crassly described it a "booger of a business meeting . . . enough to make one want to abolish the democratic system." Through it she gained new insights into the problems of the developing church in East Pakistan.

The missionaries wanted to finance a trip for the pastor to attend a conference in the Philippines. When he came before the church to ask for its endorsement, he confronted a family which opposed his leadership. Hidden feelings were exposed which later led to one of the members being physically assaulted. Mavis considered the event "a very disappointing exposure of un-Christian personality traits—my own lack of longsuffering as well. God grant me more love, more patience, more gentleness!" Though she admired the pastor's patience and "attributes of the Holy Spirit," the apparent inability of the missionaries to discipline the outbursts dismayed her.[1]

Why is it that missionaries seem to have a tendency to mollycoddle, overlook, easily forgive the national time and time again, even without repentance and request of forgiveness—sometimes apparently to the detriment of that Christian's growth. Maybe this is being slow to anger, longsuffering, and patient. God grant me more of all three! But on the other hand those same ones seem to be consistently ready to tear down, to hamper, to make unhappy, to criticize, to lessen effectiveness.

Fortunately, after the dust settled, the members reconciled. The pastor attended the conference, and Mavis exulted that, "We at the same time saw some exemplary Christian love, longsuffering, and tolerance. Won't heaven be a wonderful place?"[2]

Buoyed up by a 90 on her Bengali exam, Mavis began to anticipate the coming visit of the "big three" from the Foreign Mission Board. She hoped that Drs. Cauthen, Crawley, and Fowler could give her some definite idea about her future, whether to stay in Pakistan and await a possible change of mind concerning the hospital, begin an immunization project, or transfer to a new field. In the meantime, she busied herself interviewing new household help and instructing a Girl Scout group in first aid. She even dreamed of retirement years when she might go into the motel and service-station business with her sister Gwen. But she asked, "What am I doing planning retirement? It looks like I came to Pakistan and retired!"

In a called meeting for the East Pakistan Baptist Mission (November 2, 1966), Dr. Winston Crawley, area director for the Orient, gave a thought-provoking talk on "Rethinking the Pakistan Situation" which Mavis considered admirable. Then Dr. Baker James Cauthen, executive secretary of the Foreign Mission Board, "came alive" after an exhausting journey, to lead in a spiritual worship experience. He challenged the missionaries to live in the "now" and not to dream about the past or wish for the future. In a personal conference with Dr. Crawley, he encouraged Mavis to think about the various options open to her, mainly to stay or to think of transfer to another location in the Orient, such as Thailand, Singapore, or Hong Kong. Now was the time to consider a specific goal and a definite time schedule. Dr. Cauthen capped off the mission meeting with another stirring message on "God Is Able and Provides Sufficient Grace." Mavis found, as usual, that Gloria Thurman was her most patient and understanding sounding board after the conference.[3]

An unexpected relaxation of visa restrictions led to the thought that Mavis might stay in Pakistan for a while, in case the hospital were to be approved and the mission found itself needing a nurse. As a result, Jim McKinley, the Mission chairman, asked her if she were willing to take charge of the guest house again. Since she had served in that capacity before, Mavis agreed on condition that the mission would set definite policies regarding its operation.[4]

This time Mavis's persistence paid off. Charles Beckett met with her and the personnel committee and worked out the delegation of authority for the guest house operation. As a result of the splendid spirit she felt in the mission, she related:[5]

There is one compensation for these two or three years of being a "rolling stone." I have many new and wonderful friends. Another compensation is that I really think I have grown a little spiritually (some physically too) in that I have come to the point of really surrendering a few more things to God's way instead of my own way. You know, there are some things you just can't do yourself. Yes, that's ole diehard speaking! (from a letter of 11/13/66).

Immunization Clinics

Her determination to be used in the medical field led her to offer free immunizations to the church congregation on Wednesday nights. Mavis hoped to encourage the Christians to advertise this service to others. *Perhaps*, she thought, *in this way the idea of an immunization clinic will develop.* It was too close to Christmas to resume at the Holy Family Hospital.

Perhaps as a beginning for this new idea, or perhaps out of her continual talent for entertaining, Mavis invited one of the Pakistani Mission employees and his family for Thanksgiving dinner. She served them Bengali style in deference to his young children. Mavis offered shrimp gumbo because of its rice base which is the staple diet in the country. "I marvel at their appetites for the canned Louisiana yams, fresh cucumbers, mango sauce, fruitcake, and coffee, despite the fact that a heavy East Pakistani weighs 98 pounds wet!" as she put it. The very enjoyable day ended on a sour note for the children. She ended the session by giving cholera and typhoid shots to three of them![6]

Mavis had her first real opportunity to share her faith with a Muslim through the immunization clinics:[7]

Last week's prayer meeting was in one of the office worker's homes. He invited Muslim neighbors in to get their injection (not to prayer meeting, unfortunately) and out of the conversation with him I am going back there to give other neighbors the shots. We sat and chatted with the man thirty or forty-five minutes after the procedure of getting all his family "shot." I felt that it was one of the few real opportunities to express a reason for being here and to demonstrate the things we want to do because God is love, and He loves us. We try in like manner to show our love for Him and for others. In addition to going to Dilip's home for those clinics, I am trying to find out if some of the other Christians would like to make similar arrangements in their homes to have their neighbors receive the injections.

She discovered through this experience that medical service, coupled with a sensitive explanation of one's faith, is a means of aiding the Muslim to see that the true God is a God of love. Love motivated Mavis's service and her presentation of the gospel message. As she neared another Christmas overseas, she shared this conviction with her loved ones at home:[8]

I look to find peace in the assurance that I seek to do our Lord's will in all that I do and stay in the place that I find myself during this Christmas season.

Christmas in East Pakistan

Mavis planned to spend Christmas in Faridpur with the Carl Ryther family, to the disappointment of the church people in Dacca. But before leaving, she hosted a Christmas-tree-decorating party for the single girls at the church. She improvised a mobile tree with coat hangers, tree limbs, and popcorn strings. Her exposure to the Pakistani Christmas inspired the following description of the varieties of Christmas in Pakistan:[9]

The peace, joy, and goodwill of the Spirit of Christ will not fill the heart of many in Pakistan during this Christmas. This Christmas finds only 20,000 Christians among 55 million Muslims creating their own atmosphere to celebrate their Savior's birth. As Christ stands at the door of Pakistan and knocks, what does He see within?

In a Muslim's home (over 99 percent of all homes) it is not an ordinary day. Baba (father) is home, free of duty today, but he will go to the mosque for prayers at noon and to the stadium to hear the speeches in the afternoon. It is a holiday to commemorate the birth of Mohammed Ali Jinnah, one of the founding fathers of the nation's independence.

In the home of a Muslim converted to Christianity, . . . Elias looks at his wife and nine-month-old son with some uneasiness. His father, a Mollavi (Muslim religious teacher) and brother have been dropping in more frequently of late. They openly express the feeling that he belongs with them back in the Muslim home and culture and would consider it their duty to take him there. A new sari on his wife, a vivid green karilyn (synthetic fiber) suit on his son, and his own dazzling white punjabi are the Christmas gifts of this household. At 9 a.m. he will direct the opening of the special Christmas worship service. He is the assistant pastor of Immanuel Church.

In a Hindu convert's home . . . A one-room rented house with thatch walls, there are three crepe-paper decorations and a beautiful calendar picture of Christ in the place of honor. The four children are proudly dressed in this year's only new clothes . . . Baba is leaving early for church. He is the custodian and usher, a radiant Christian. He has made arrangements for the feast and will be standing by with a gracious and confident smile, ready to help any and all.

In a third-generation Christian's home . . . The meager furnishings of their first home make this a mansion for him and his Christian bride of six months. Twisted crepe paper and a crepe-paper bell decorate it. During this year he has completed law exams, attended the Asia Youth Conference, and made preparations to begin three years' study at the Baptist Seminary in the Philippines. He kneels in prayer and in preparation for this Christmas Day. This is his first Christmas as pastor and today, as all other days, he will preach Christ dynamically.

In a Baptist Church . . . Colorful and sparkling saris "decorate" the women's side of the auditorium as the predominant white of the men's punjabis seems to reflect the glow from the other side. Men, women, and children left their shoes at the door, an unseasonable custom, and sit gracefully and comfortably on straw mats. Crepe-paper decorations hang from every available spot and may adorn the building for months to come. Every night during this past week, the young people met at different homes for a "kirtone" (hymn-sing) and fellowship. Again at daybreak this morning they awoke many Christian families with their song. Last evening, just at dark, there was pageantry and inspiration in the candle-lighting ceremony. After all candles were lit, an old beggar-man appeared with token gifts for all the children. It was Father Christmas sent by the Sunday School! Today, as soon as the worship service is over, the congregation will go to the mission house for the love feast. There will be the warm sharing as all pitch in to prepare the chicken curry, rice and roshogollas (a sweet). It will also be one of the highlights of the year for most of the participants. Later this afternoon there will be a Christmas drama done by the students of the Mission Industrial School.

In a missionary's home . . . During the season, the pastor and his wife and another Bengali couple were invited for a holiday dinner. Some nursing and medical students, including a Muslim student, shared a holiday meal. There was an "Open House" for the Mission family, and there was a night of caroling from the roof with the Sisters from the local Catholic hospital. Probably the best of all was sewing some scraps of material for some little girl's Christmas attire and improvising Christmas decorations from the things at hand. The chicken-and-dressing Christmas dinner was last night, leaving today for the Love Feast. The wonderfully packable aluminum tree is the "touch of home" that glistens above the fold-up manger scene like so many stars over Bethlehem. The sparkling and jingling tree ornaments made of tin-can tops saved from last year's larder attracts the attention of many passing the front gate. With the crisp sweater-sleeve weather, the recorded Christmas carols in the air, the tree . . . is this America or Pakistan?

In some ways Christmas in Pakistan is the same. In the sanctuary of the Universal Church there is the same choir of the heavenly hosts, the same brotherly love, the same shepherds! In the Kingdom of God there is the same King of kings and Lord of lords!

Amid new insights following the short time in Nepal, Mavis began to "lean on the Lord" more. As a result she shared, "I'll make it in the coming months because of the promise so beautifully expressed in this poem by Amy Lively":

God Sees

God sees around the corner
Just where I cannot see.
He sees around the corner
And knows what's there for me.
A blank wall is before me,
Blank walls on either side;
The gate is closed behind me;
There is no place to hide.
But I know there is a corner
That yet I cannot see.
God knows that 'round that corner
Is just what's best for me.

Mavis did not find it easy to commit the future to the Lord, but she tried. "Needless to tell you, all is not peaceful inside, but I can most of the time leave the situation in God's hands. I trust that soon I will be able to dig into some work with a little substance to it and can gripe about being too busy for a while."[11] The New Year ushered in new activities but not the final word about the future.

A touching letter from her pastor repaid Mavis's generosity in joining with fellow missionaries to send him to the Third Asian Baptist Youth Conference:

The gift you have given me this year in the way of financing for the Philippines conference was a presentation of genuine worth. It has brought many blessings into my life to deepen substantially my understanding as a laborer in the kingdom of God.

On looking back, I always find a feeling of gratitude to you all for the genuine, tender, and warm assistance much more generously than I always deserved. The way you have known my need to have a job after my father's death, the arrangement of bringing me to Dacca for studies, my keen interest in a conference like the one I attended, has shown your unfailing sympathy and kindness to me and my family. Once again I convey my thanks to you all with a grateful and humble heart.

I felt the need to dedicate my life in the conference for the year of 1967. I received wonderful peace in such dedication.

Lastly, I do not have anything to give you in remembrance of your help and love to me, yet I promise that my thoughts, my works, my activities will submissively pay their regards to you now and ever.

Gloria Thurman's arrival in Dacca compounded Mavis's joy of having shared in the training of her pastor. Gloria was expecting her first child and Mavis anxiously anticipated being present to greet him or her into the world! With clinical detail Mavis recorded the whole birth procedure in her diary and entered that at precisely 2:37 A.M. on January 7, 1967, "Philip Edward here!" Mavis called Tom at 4:00 a.m. and greeted him with, "Good morning, Father Tom!" Mavis had never seen a first delivery so uncomplicated. Tom was "happy and grateful" and Gloria was "radiant and recuperating fast. Such a fine, mature Christian couple." Mavis doted over "my" baby for the few days in the hospital and noted that he is "7 lbs. 10 oz. and 22 inches in length, a very good baby—started on cereal the first night." A letter from Gloria rewarded Mavis's "tender, loving care" for the Thurmans:

Wednesday night, January 11, 1967

Dear Mavis,

As I thought back over the past few days, I once again realized how much you have done for us. I can truthfully say that I had no "uneasiness" Friday night, because I felt assured that you knew how to handle the situation. And you did! 'Twas a big boost to me to have you standing by in the delivery room. Perhaps your important role of the night was letting the father know. I appreciate your willingness to "tackle the operator" at that time of day.

Eye-Openers

Plans to take a boat from Khulna to the Sunderbans did not work out. The delay necessitated spending the night in the home of British Baptist missionaries in this booming mill town in the middle of the southern marshlands. Mavis had not appreciated sufficiently the high standard of support afforded to missionaries of the Southern Baptist Convention until she saw how these other colleagues lived.[13]

They were ever so hospitable but just didn't have the conveniences and the privileges we do . . . No screens, no mosquito nets, crude furnishings, and strictly living from the local market. Not that we suffered, but we didn't sleep as well as usual, and we were made more conscious of the things we have that are not absolute necessities. Nonetheless, they certainly make life more comfortable and we remembered to be very grateful to the Lottie Moon Christmas Offerings which make it possible for us to have those comforts.

Travel for foreigners in East Pakistan is always an adventure. Crowds gathered continually to gawk at strange white people and their unfamiliar mannerisms.

The first day we didn't feel up to the crowds so we ate in the car while traveling. The second day we were braver and stopped by the roadside to eat. Only some twenty-five or thirty gathered by the time we finished eating. That is one of the most difficult things for me to accept—the unabashed staring of the people. It is almost impossible to intimidate them into leaving. They just simply stop, make themselves comfortable, and stare!

Charles Beckett once asked Mavis, "Do the men and their constant staring intimidate you?" She balled up her fist and said, "If I could handle those big sailors on the ship *Hope*, I can certainly handle these little Pakistani men!"

Arriving back in Dacca she found correspondence piled up in the guest house and the gardener on leave to get married. Her reflections on this reveal a bit of her own feelings on the subject of marriage and her empathy for the people she served:[14]

We have another wedding in the "family." The lady who works for me had to have time off to go back to her village and bring her daughter to Dacca. She is going to give her in marriage to the gardener who works here. The girl is around sixteen years old, and he must be thirty or more—no doubt on her way to a house full of kids and early widowhood. It is beyond understanding to see these people without enough to eat but to whom the most important thing in the world is to have as many children as possible. I am grateful that I have the opportunity to forego marriage bliss if I so chose! No bitterness—but there are some things that are worse.

East Pakistan, with a population of over 63,000,000 in 1967, was one of the most densely populated countries in the world. In a land area slightly larger than Mavis's native state of Louisiana, American aid officials rated the population density at 1,100 per square mile, among the world's highest![15] Muslim teaching against birth control led to a population growth of over 3 percent per year. At a maternity shower Mavis gave these statistics—"Every hour in East Pakistan there are 14,000 babies being born." Her simplistic remedy was, "Since family planning is one of our projects, it is our job to find those women and stop them!"[16] Despite the humorous way she viewed the need for birth control she was not unaware of infant mortality. "You do not count chickens around here even after they hatch. It is a fact that most of the people do not name their babies until they are at least one year old because the infant death rate is so high!"[17]

The Baptist Mission celebrated its tenth anniversary in East Pakistan on February 7, 1967. It was a joyous occasion with a chalk-talk devotional in the afternoon on "Who Am I?" and a fun time reminiscing to the tune of "Three Blind Mice." Mavis appeared in a space suit to indicate the direction for the future. Then there was a reading on "If the next ten years are like the first ten, will we make it?" An unforeseen event on the way home turned the light-hearted frolic into sober reality.

About five miles out of Faridpur a little girl darted in front of the car. The driver's quick reaction could not prevent her being hit. After the car rolled to a stop, Mavis, to her relief, found that the girl suffered only a broken leg. They quickly gathered up the child and her mother and hurried to the nearest hospital where the doctors recommended she be taken to Dacca for better treatment. The family consented to the girl's treatment and settled the case to the satisfaction of all parties. But it was a shocking reminder for Mavis and the other missionaries that one of the greatest dangers in overseas service is not from war or political uprisings but on the highways.

Mavis herself gained a reputation for being a tenacious driver. Dacca is a city of unbelievable traffic congestion where bicycle taxis, buses, automobiles, and pedestrians all vie for the right-of-way while driving British style on the left-hand side of the road. Gloria Thurman remembers Mavis's stubbornness behind the wheel:[18]

The most frightened I have ever been was while riding in Dacca. Mavis was driving. Most local drivers take their half of the road right down the middle. Mavis drove a small VW. She would pull right to the center lane line and stop (on her side of the road). The driver coming toward her would eventually pull over to his lane just before there was a headon crash!

The traffic in Karachi, West Pakistan, added an unexpected dimension. Mavis flew there with Dr. Jeanne Beckett to check on getting reciprocity and registration for doctors and nurses. "A most amazing and different thing to me are the camels and camel carts. The first time I've ever seen them outside of a zoo!"[19] Pakistani traffic was not the only challenge Mavis faced.

Loneliness

In mid-March 1967, Mavis found herself faced again with the dilemma of her future as a missionary nurse in East Pakistan. Would the government ever give permission to build the hospital? Little did she or others know that behind the government's stalling of the project were forces beyond anyone's control.

Eid Al-Adha, the feast of the sacrifice, arrived again, and all the other missionaries had left town. Mavis felt lonely. Loneliness plagues single missionaries and all who leave family, home, and familiar surroundings. Her indecision about the future exacerbated the loneliness, as she indicated in her diary:

Which way, Lord? I feel no clear leading in any direction but feel I *need* the contacts of the medical conference (in Hong Kong) very much. Maybe the direction is to be found there. Just received a letter from Rosemary (Spessard) to come to Thailand and help train five nurses for OR. Good news to be wanted and needed. Will go to Hong Kong and see.

Loneliness increased when she realized she would never be able to satisfy the expectations of the nationals among whom she worked. Minor matters, such as being responsible for a mimeograph machine and having to refuse its use to others, became a burden to her:[20]

I did not have the authority to give them permission to use the machine. My name is now "dirty missionary." It is so true that the Eastern mind just does not function like the Western mind, and I'm beginning to believe the "twain ne'er shall meet!"

Later her unexpected trip to Karachi meant that she missed church in Dacca. This oversight caused her anguish, as indicated in a letter home:[22]

That's better than going to church when you make three mad because you didn't go by their house and wait 30 minutes so they could go with you. You make five mad because they can't ride home with you. You make three mad because you didn't stay home to be asked about using the duplicating machine. Three more are unhappy because you didn't come by last week to tell them you were going to Karachi (on two days' notice) and wouldn't be by to pick them up on Sunday! Bitter! Who me? Never! Just stating the facts, man! *Don't ever let anyone know that we have got human beings over here too!!* As I understand it we ain't supposed to be this sinful (Ha!).

Love you, Bill

The morale of the fellow missionaries also concerned her. She saw how happy they were with each visa that was approved, and she saw how spirits were lifted when they heard of a couple returning to the field. For her it indicated "what my leaving might do to morale!"[23] All this combined with an attack of amoebic dysentery found her in March 1967 with a "great depression in the Bay of Pate."[24] As the plane lifted off the runway to Hong Kong and a medical conference, she hoped the depression would leave!

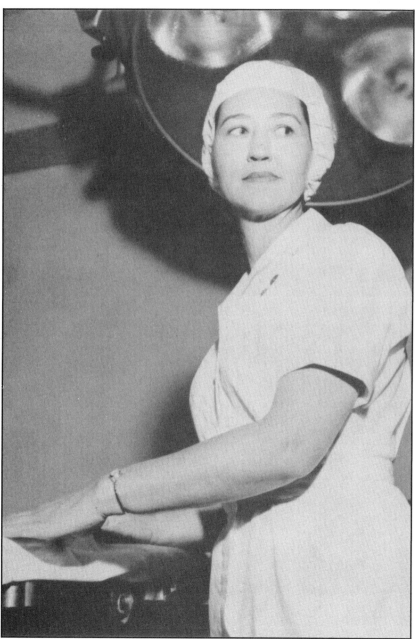

Mavis Orisca Pate, R.N., (as she was shown on the cover of *Diary of Hope*) was operating room supervisor on the *S. S. Hope* in 1960–61. Ethicon, Incorporated, commissioned Pate to write the book (© Copyright, Ethicon, Inc., 1962. Picture used by permission.).

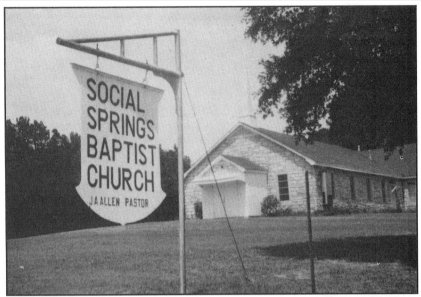

Social Springs Baptist Church, Mavis's home church, which figured prominently in her acceptance of Christ and His call to service.

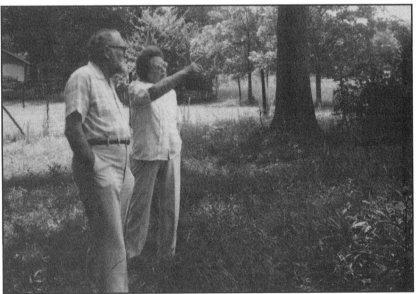

Mavis's mother and her pastor at Mavis's "praying tree" (Photos courtesy of the Pate family).

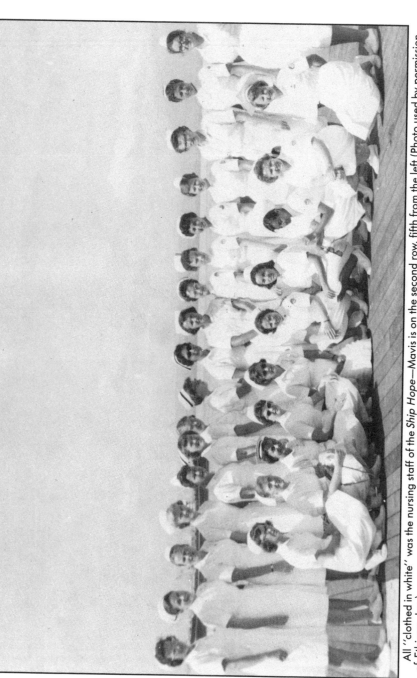

All "clothed in white" was the nursing staff of the *Ship Hope*—Mavis is on the second row, fifth from the left (Photo used by permission of Ethicon, Inc.).

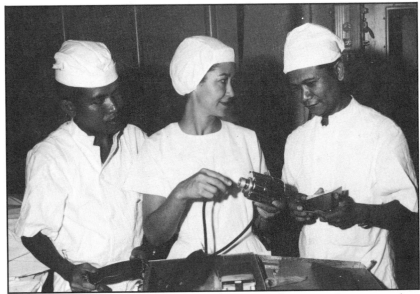

Mavis demonstrating equipment and procedures to Indonesian male nurses on the *S. S. Hope* (Photo used by permission of Ethicon, Inc.).

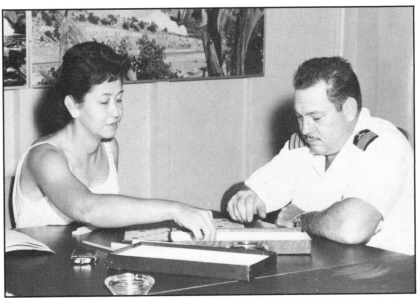

Mavis and *Hope* Chief Engineer Charles Strobaker (United States Information Service Photograph, Djakarta, Indonesia).

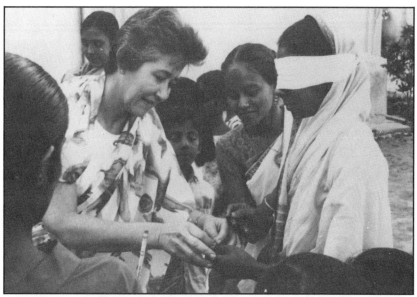

Missionary Mavis Pate playing a game with women and children at a party in Bangladesh. Mavis was popular wherever God led her because of her talent for creating fun.

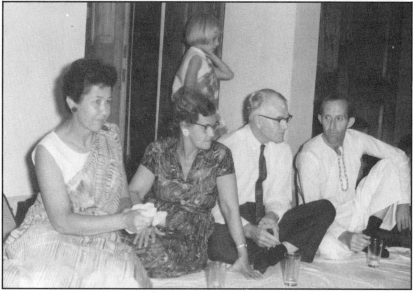

Missionary Pate, a lay couple (in middle), and Missionary Jim McKinley enjoyed a meal in a Bangladesh missionary residence (Both Foreign Mission Board, SBC, Photos by Moore).

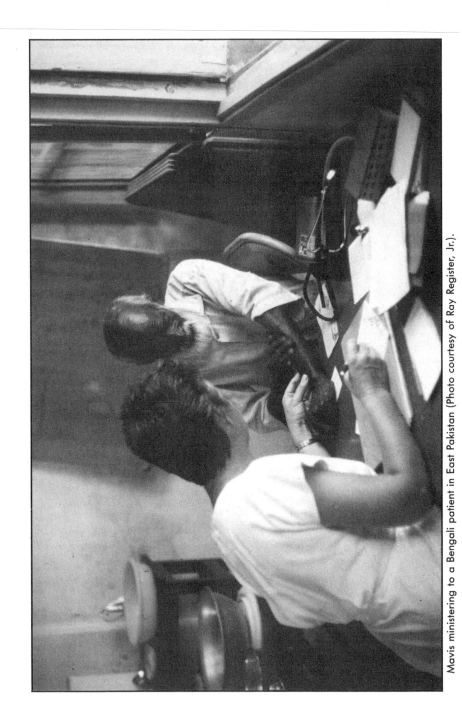

Mavis ministering to a Bengali patient in East Pakistan (Photo courtesy of Ray Register, Jr.).

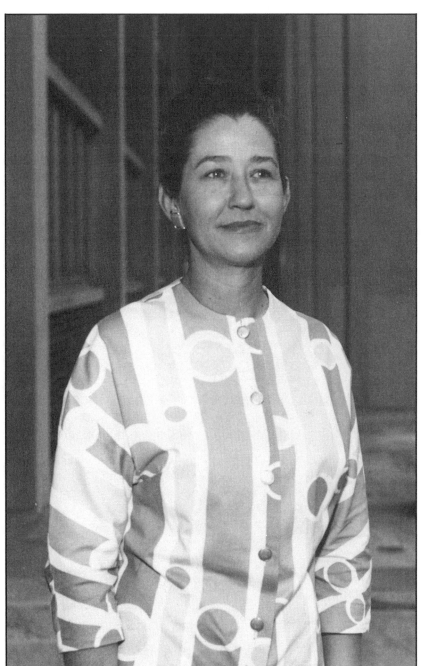

Mavis posed for this portrait right after she was appointed missionary to East Pakistan on July 16, 1964 (Foreign Mission Board Photo by Snedden).

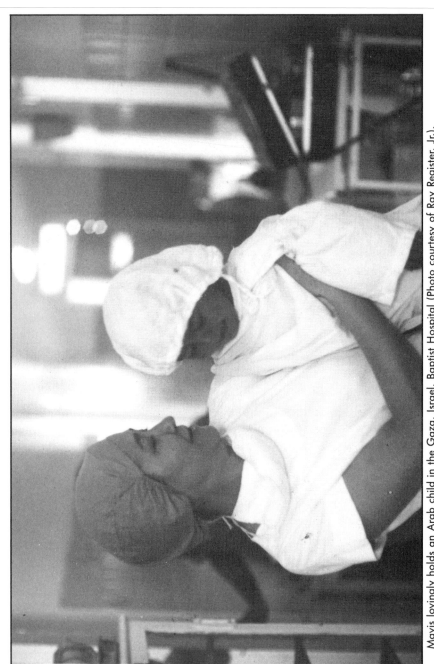

Mavis lovingly holds an Arab child in the Gaza, Israel, Baptist Hospital (Photo courtesy of Ray Register, Jr.).

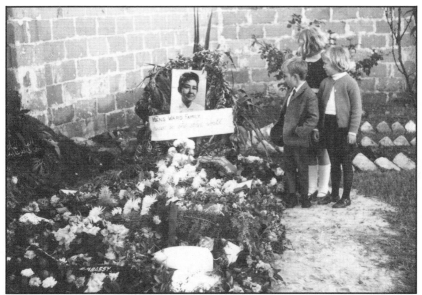

MKs Mellisa Moore, Cary Peach, and Davis Peach at Mavis's graveside (Photo Courtesy of Ray Register, Jr.).

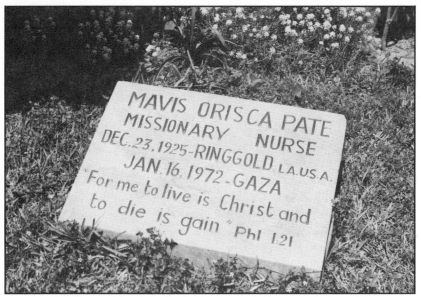

MAVIS ORISCA PATE
MISSIONARY   NURSE
DEC. 23, 1925 - RINGGOLD, LA. US. A.
JAN. 16, 1972 - GAZA
"For me to live is Christ and
to die is gain" Phl 1.21

Mavis had requested that if she died on the mission field, that she be buried there. Her wish was carried out. Her grave is on the grounds of Ahli Arab Hospital, formerly Baptist Hospital (Foreign Mission Board Photo by Scofield).

7

East Pakistan: Part III

Hong Kong

Her trip to Hong Kong temporarily pulled Mavis out of her depression. As she talked with Everly Hayes, Ruth Austin, and Dr. Ralph Bethea from Indonesia she learned of many places that needed nurses in established medical work. But they always conditioned the advice, "If it's God's will." Dr. Bethea seemed to discourage her moving since he didn't want to proselytize Pakistan's nurses. He felt they should pray for the government to change its mind about the hospital. She shared her thoughts with Earl Goatcher over lunch. He advised, "Mavis, don't be afraid to do 180 degrees!"[1]

Squeezed in between sessions at the medical conference, Mavis talked twice with Dr. Winston Crawley. The first session she received information and prayed about opportunities. In a letter written from Hong Kong on April 7, 1967, to her family, she shared the outcome of her thoughts:

The past few days were difficult ones for me. The struggle of searching out God's will continued until about the middle of yesterday afternoon. Then I was like the dove who was sent out from Noah's Ark. I couldn't find dry land on which to put my feet so I returned home! It was not that no other fields needed a nurse. They all did and had invited me to come, but nothing seemed right *or* my "dish." I will return to Pakistan and write a letter immediately asking for transfer out of Dacca to Comilla (The closest vacant residence to Dr. Jeanne Beckett). I will begin the second-year language study, will "open me a clinic," and will accept any request from other fields for short-term help in my "specialty."

Love, Bill

Sometime in the afternoon of April 6, Mavis made her decision to remain in East Pakistan. Her "180-degree" decision returned her to that difficult Muslim land. That evening Dr. Crawley's message on "Love as the Motive of Missions" registered in Mavis's heart. After the meeting Mavis fellowshipped with Dora Howard, Bill and Bob Wakefield, Troy Bennett, Charles Beckett, and Jim McKinley, all stalwarts of Southeast Asian missions. On the way back to the hotel Mavis and Jim talked. She said, "Regardless of what happens about the hospital in East Pakistan, I'm going to stay here. I can find some way to serve the Lord." That night Dora became like a sister, and the men like brothers who cared enough to share in this difficult decision. Mavis established a new relationship to the East Pakistan mission and received renewed hope for the future.

She shared her decision with Dr. Crawley a few days later at the Kowloon Baptist Church. He agreed to it with an understanding on which she depended. She left with a much lighter heart.

Muharram

Back in Dacca, Mavis found the populace in the holiday spirit. Bengali Muslims celebrated "Muharram." A long-awaited barrel arrived from the States, putting Mavis in a festive mood. Without any premonition of the future she shared her Hong Kong experiences in a letter home telling of the many opportunities for nursing in the Orient and adding as an aside, "And then there is the Gaza Strip Hospital." Little did she realize, at the time, how much this aside would cost her one day!

The rainy season arrived in late April 1967. Mavis busied herself sewing an A-line dress and a "laundry bag" shift dress for her next stint in Bogra to assist Dr. Fidelia Gilbert at the Church of God Mission Hospital. She oriented Dora on the operation of the guest house and how to care for Gretchen, her dachshund dog. This was a special order since Gretchen loved peanut brittle and bananas almost as much as the MKs that frequented Mavis' apartment!

Mavis was anxious to "pick Dr. Gilbert's brains" for guidance about her work in the future. Then she hoped to visit the Catholic leprosarium and an Australian Baptist medical establishment in the Northeast part of the country. She also planned to continue her second year in Bengali language study. But she secretly questioned if she had the self-discipline to improve her broken Bengali.

Back to Bogra

Pastor Biswas met Mavis at the train station in Bogra. The flame tree in view from Mavis's room showed its lovely scarlet flowers in contrast to the filth and squalor of the town. Any trip to town earned Mavis "the stares, the comments one doesn't have to know the language to understand, the honest curiosity, and the inevitable crowd that collects and accompanies one to each place on the route."[3]

Mavis quickly plunged into the first "real work" she had done for a year, taking life histories in her broken Bengali, learning to do examinations, and the like. She soon got to the "I'll-explode-if-I-hear-one-more-Bengali-word" stage.

Hospital service led to invitations into the homes of Muslim friends providing eye-openers into the local customs:[5]

Last Thursday Hothim (first name) Babu (honorific name) and his family invited Dr. Gilbert and me to dinner. When we arrived we went into an area of the house separated from the menfolk and were left by ourselves part of the time, and the ladyfolk talked with us part of the time. When the meal was ready, we found the two of us seated with the male guest and the son of the family while the lady of the house, her teenaged daughter, and her husband stood by to talk and serve. Sometimes no member of the household eats with the guests. And in the true Muslim culture, I think the custom is that no ladies eat until the men have eaten. In the most strict Muslim homes, I think the lady of the house is never seen but only comes out to greet the guests and disappears for the remainder of the time. Of course, in such cultures there are probably no lady guests.

The deeper exposure to Bengali culture caused Mavis to reflect humorously on the difference from Western etiquette and male-female relationships:[5]

> Let no man deceive himself. If any man among you seemeth to be wise in this world, let him become a fool, that he may be wise (1 Cor. 3:18, KJV).

For how many years I went through the process (sometimes torment)of getting myself educated and adding a little cultural refinement. *And lo!* Now I am back to eating with my fingers, and I must furnish my own utensils if I must use them (but that is in reality rather unrefined!). The way to serve is apparently the shortest distance between two points—stand up if you can't reach what you need sitting down. Now I have learned it is considerate if you leave soon after the meal, if you crack the chicken bones for the marrow, and if you belch loudly in appreciation!

Women are not expected to know enough to talk with men, besides they must be protected from the man beast. A woman on a train struck up a conversation with Dr. Gilbert sometime in the past. She asked her in amazement and sheer disbelief if Dr. Gilbert was traveling alone? Dr. Gilbert assured her she was. After a pause to gaze upon this unbelievable creature, the woman asked, "Are you afraid of men?" Dr. Gilbert said, "No." Then she asked, "Are you afraid of a tiger?" Dr. Gilbert said, "Yes." Then the woman confided, "I'm more afraid of men than I am a tiger!"

The contrast of cultures provoked Mavis to consider her own role in life:

Maybe that very pride and vanity in feeling a little indispensable and necessary at my job (and making it my whole life) was something from which I needed to be weaned. I told God I was willing to be made willing to do His will. Maybe He is still "making" me. This is not at all said in bitterness. Rather a little in awe of God's ways, a little wistful of many ifs, ands and buts, and much in humor with the ways of man and the universe.

The time in Bogra passed quickly. Mavis headed back to Dacca through the lush forested area of Myansingh where the Catholics had a leprosarium. She stopped for a visit.

For a Louisiana nurse who had never been to the leprosarium at Carville in her home state,[6] Mavis sure got around! As soon as she arrived back to the bustle of Dacca she was off again to a tour of duty in Bangkla, Thailand![7]

Busy in Bangkla

Rode out to Bangkla next day with Dr. Butcher. The Oklahoma Baptist University Choir on S.E. Asian Tour was in Bangkla for concert and supper . . . I have had time for at least two hours class each day. Class does not move too fast through an interpreter! Dr. Rebekah Ann Naylor is here on a Smith-Kline-French Fellowship, a drug company that sponsors senior medical students in a mission hospital for ten weeks experience.

It is a little ego-pleasing to return where I have labored before. I see some results of the previous efforts and it is gratifying to know all is not in vain. It is amazing what can be done with grammar-school graduates when it is necessary. This little "one-hoss" town hospital has the appearance of a twenty-five bed intensive care unit. It is good to get my fingernails and my elbows clean again!!

The same commitment to heal people's bodies and spirits, which drew Mavis to the mission field, continued to radiate from the Bangkla Baptist Hospital as she indicated in a newsletter on August 29, 1967:

This hospital may not have a cure for the cancer that tortures their bodies but they have compassion. And they have peace for the soul which is offered to all. This week there were admitted to the hospital, among others, a family of six with malaria, a 19-year-old girl who lost her hand in a windmill, two men infected with anthrax when they butchered a cow, a young girl for an appendectomy, and a mother to deliver her firstborn. These have all heard the gospel preached and music that proclaimed God's love. They have heard the personal witnessing of mission doctors, nurses, and of Thai Christians.

Dr. Joann Goatcher led a couple's week-day Bible study class. Last Easter eleven members of that class were baptized. "Christians are the only people who will visit us here," say the patients in the Leprosy-T.B. Rehabilitation Building. Thai young men and women are trained here as nurse's assistants. Three of the last class of twelve, originally from Buddhist homes, accepted Christ as their Savior and now they tell others too. The pastor of the newly organized Bangkla Baptist Church spent seven years as a Buddhist priest before becoming a Christian five years ago.

Unexpected news from Pakistan helped Mavis's mind to stand the sweltering heat that September. The mission approved an early furlough because of visa and work distribution considerations. That meant going home in 1968 rather than 1969.

Afghanistan

The East Pakistan mission "family" met Mavis at the Dacca airport when she returned from Thailand. Her new downstairs neighbors for the few months before furlough were the Howard Teels. For the umpteenth time, she tried to whip up enthusiasm for Bengali study, but her mind wandered to the trip home and her plans to visit the Holy Land. After a mission retreat at Cox's Bazaar she decided to accompany Dora Howard on a vacation to West Pakistan and Afghanistan. A letter home after they returned on December 9, 1967, describes the fun they had:

Back in Dacca again! It was a great trip. I'll give the rundown on places seen just so you'll know we didn't drag our feet on the way. Not even when we rode in those horse-drawn "tongas" on only two wheels with what appeared to be a delicate balance between the front and the back. Reminds me of the ones in the islands of Indonesia when we would lift the horses off the ground when getting into the thing from the front!

Mon. Nov. 27- Left Dacca for Lahore, West Pakistan. Stayed there two nights and in our sightseeing we found some marble carvings that we wanted to do "temple rubbings" of. With some fast talking, we got to do two the next morning. We could not leave without completing them so that sort of set the pattern for our departure from each place. We raced to make the plane because we found our opportunities to do rubbings at the eleventh hour.

Nov. 29th- Left Lahore for Rawalpindi. We had no answers from our letters of about three weeks before requesting reservations so we had to find a place to stay in each city. We stayed in the first motel to be opened in Pakistan. A very homey and restful atmosphere with open fireplace. It was cold. We took a mini-bus and went to see Islamabad, the newly constructed capital city of Pakistan.

Nov. 30th- Went on to Peshawar in northern West Pakistan. This city is in the foothills of the mountains, cool and invigorating. Only problem was that to read a book in the room we had to go to bed under two blankets, with sweater and gloves! No heat in the rooms. We looked over the city and made arrangements for our visas and trip to Afghanistan. Didn't find anything to "rub" on the first trip.

Dec. 2- By bus over the Khyber Pass, we went to Kabul the capital of Afghanistan. We went to church twice on Sunday at the American Community Church and had lunch with Christy Wilson, pastor of the church, and with Dr. Bob Bucher from Iran. They showed us Baba er-Baba's tomb with marble carvings to "rub" which kept us busy Monday and Tuesday.

Dec. 5- Returned to Peshawar by plane. We visited the English Mission Hospital and found some beautiful wood carvings in their chapel to "rub."

Dec. 6- Flew back to Rawalpindi and decided to spend the remaining time in the homey motel with the fireplace. No luck in finding anything to rub so we went shopping and bought a wood carving to bring home and rub.

Dec. 8- Arrived in Dacca about 7:30 P.M. Gotta get in high gear to get packing done, go to school, and get ready for Christmas.

Love to each and all,

Bill

Packing

Back in Dacca time passed quickly at the guest house as Mavis received a steady stream of visitors for the Christmas season. She busily prepared a drum of mementos to ship to the States for her furlough. In the midst of the activities her cook brought her an unexpected guest:

Just had a memorable guest. It was the mother of my helper. He came as excited as could be telling me his mother was in his quarters and was coming to see me. She was a very country lady, and I could hardly understand her Bengali—can't understand much at best. She had on a sari, pink with orange border, that may be the latest combination but there was something clashing about it. Bernard's little sister was with her. She was ten years old. I served them tea and cookies and then Bernard said she wanted to see my house and things so I showed them all through. It was embarrassing in a way. All seven of her children and she and her husband probably live in a house about the size of my living room and here I am—one person in a six-room house and two bathrooms! (from a letter of 1/14/68).

Unexpected news also broke! Dora Howard and W. L. Loftland announced their plans to be married on March 12. Mavis was happy, but disappointed that she would miss the wedding:[10]

This wedding is really going to be the social event of the year. Dora has decided to wear a silk sari and Gloria, as her matron of honor, will wear a blue one. Next to the Vietnamese dress, I think the sari is the prettiest woman's dress I have seen. The wedding will be in the ballroom at the Intercontinental Hotel and Dr. Crawley who is coming into Dacca for about twenty-four hours will perform the ceremony.

Half her mission "family" appeared at the Dacca airport to see Mavis off on Monday, March 4, 1968. As she settled back on the flight to Teheran via Karachi, she wondered what unanticipated adventures lay ahead in the Holy Land.

The Holy Land

An impressive tour highlighted her overnight stop in Teheran. She saw it all: Sepahsalr Mosque, Golestan Palace and the National Bank Vault containing the crown jewels, and the peacock throne. Mavis reflected on the social and economic progress of Iran, and that in earlier days Cyrus the Great allowed the Jews to return from exile to Jerusalem where she would soon be. As Air France flight 197 winged over the barren hills of northern Iran and Lake Urmia, then out over the Mediterranean, excitement welled up in her heart. Mavis had become a world traveler and a "utility woman" who filled in the gaps.

Ava Nell McWhorter met Mavis at the Tel Aviv airport. They knew each other from Shreveport, Louisiana. Ava Nell instructed nursing there before appointment as a missionary nurse to the Gaza Baptist Hospital. They had attended Training Union together at the Highland Baptist Church. After an overnight at the home of Baptist Representatives, Marcus and Ruth Reed, they drove to Baptist Village Camp and Conference Center, nestled on a bend of the Yarkon River on the Sharon Plain. Bob and Eddie Fields, Milton and Marty Murphy, directors of the Center, and Journeyman Bob Dawkins greeted her and talked about the work of the former George W. Truett Orphanage.

Mavis was unaware of the apprehensive stares of Jewish Israelis, as they drove north along the ancient "Stella Maris," the "way of the sea." The tell-tale grey license plate of their Gaza car gave them away. As they arrived at the ruins of Meggido in view of the valley of Israel, the "Armageddon" of the Book of Revelation, Mavis was enthralled. Up the Galilee mountains into Nazareth, she oohed and ahed at the mosaics and ruins in the Roman Catholic Church of the Annunciation. Past the little Baptist Church at Mary's Well, they wound their way down the mountains through Cana of Galilee to Tiberias on the shores of the Sea of Galilee. As the evening lights from the villages sparkled in the hills overlooking the sea, Mavis felt a secure peace warm her heart, almost as if she had truly come home.

Early the next morning, she and Ava Nell drove north around the sea. Just before Magdala, they stopped at a picturesque spot owned by the YMCA, and Mavis waded in the Sea of Galilee. They drove on around the Mount of Beatitudes, and then to Capernaum. Standing in the ruins of the ancient synagogue, Mavis imagined she heard the words of Jesus spoken there: "I am the bread of life; he who comes to me shall not hunger, and he who believes in me shall never thirst."[11] The ruins testified to Jesus' prophecy of Capernaum's destruction because of their unbelief.

Driving south by Mount Tabor, the traditional sight of the trans-figuration, they circled into the hills of Samaria. The imposing mountains of Ebal and Gerizim rose up on both sides as they drove through the modern Arab city of Nablus to Jerusalem. As the Holy City came into view that afternoon, Mavis and Ava Nell spontaneously broke out into singing the stirring anthem "Jerusalem." Mavis had difficulty distinguishing between the ancient and the modern in its crowded landscape. After lunch and shopping at the Baptist Bookstore in East Jerusalem, they settled in for a much-needed rest at the American Colony Hotel.

The next morning, Mavis and Ava Nell made the pilgrimage to the Garden Tomb. Then they drove up to the Mount of Olives with its spectacular view of the Old City and the Golden Gate still awaiting the Second Coming of the Messiah. Visiting the Garden of Gethsemene and Caiaphas's house at the Church of the Cock Crow gave Mavis an overwhelming sense of the Lord's sufferings.

Checking out of the hotel, they headed south towards Bethlehem and the Shepherds Field. The closeness of the holy sites surprised Mavis! In less than an hour, they passed the mammoth mosque over Abraham's tomb in Hebron and dropped out of the hills of Judea onto the flat plains of Beersheba. Winter rains had fed the parched earth, and rolling hills of newly sprouted grain stretched to the horizon. In less than two hours from Jerusalem, they passed Ashkelon and soon pulled up to the Israeli border post entering the Gaza Strip. The guard recognized the Baptist Hospital car and motioned it past lines of Arab cars and trucks waiting to be searched. Mavis heaved a sigh of relief as she remembered the long weeks of waiting for permits to enter border areas in East Pakistan!

The Gaza Strip was different from what Mavis expected. Since she had heard for many years about the situation in Israel and the Arab countries, the lush orange groves on either side of the highway surprised her. *The Arabs have cared for their land after all*, she thought. She passed an American-owned bottling company and an orange packing plant. The small shops and garages reminded her somewhat of East Pakistan. Soon they pulled up to a large iron gate. Ava Nell gave a toot on the horn, and an Arab watchman swung open the gate. Inside the Gaza Baptist Hospital grounds, Mavis found herself in another world. A complex of yellow stucco buildings nestled among palm and eucalyptus trees. The high walls closed out the din of horns and noise from the street in this welcomed haven.

The hospital staff awaited Mavis's arrival. It was common knowledge that Mavis was open to a transfer to another field because of the Pakistani government's failure to grant permission to build the new hospital. She and Ava Nell corresponded about the possibility of a move. Pat Hale, newly arrived special project nurse from South Carolina, noted:[12]

We had many visitors in Gaza. Visitors who were tourists from the U.S.A. and other countries, doctors, military people, families of fellow missionaries, and also missionaries from other countries, but Mavis was special because she was coming to look us over and decide if she would apply for a transfer. Everyone was eagerly anticipating her visit. At last the day of her arrival came.

Pat had duty in the obstetrics ward when Mavis arrived, so she gave only a brief hello. But the next morning Ava Nell invited her along to show Mavis the Egyptian border town of Al Arish. On the two-hour drive south through the Sinai desert mute testimony to the 1967 war was everywhere:[13]

We arrived in El Arish and parked our car. As we walked along the deserted sandy beach we saw evidences of war and fighting. There were burned-out jeeps and trucks on the beach and also a train that had been burned. The town was almost deserted. This made all of us very sad to realize the devastation that existed as a result of the fighting.

The somber mood of the group changed upon returning to Gaza. Mavis donned her sari for tea with the mission staff and showed slides of Pakistan. She laughed as they compared the difficulty of learning the Arabic and Bengali languages. Mavis enjoyed the company of Dr. David Dorr and his wife, Roberta. She felt affirmed by Dr. Merrill Moore and Patty Moore. Her hosts, Jim and Betty Smith, were on loan from Ashkelon, Israel, while Chaplain Ed and Anne Nicholas were on furlough. Meeting these and the missionary nursing staff caused her to wonder if they would play a future role in her life.

Mavis arose early on Sunday morning to attend the Arab church service. She noted the kneeling benches in the former Episcopal church as Pastor Ibrahim Hanna spoke. Occasionally she recognized a word similar to Bengali. After a tour of the hospital compound, the personnel drove Mavis and Pat Hale out to the crossroad near Ashkelon to catch a bus to Jerusalem. It was Pat's first visit to the Holy City. The next day they made a memorable visit to the Garden Tomb:

I well remember Mavis commenting on our visit there that this place seemed to mean the most to her. While there we took time to find a quiet place in the garden to meditate and thank God for His Son Jesus who really did rise from the dead in a spot near to us and from a tomb similar to this one. I thanked Him again that the tomb was empty. Indeed it had been a memorable day, spent with Mavis on my first trip to Jerusalem.[14]

Early on Tuesday, March 12, 1968, Mavis left the Lod Airport on a flight to Athens. A short tour of the historic Greek city and a later stop in London could not drive the indelible impressions of Gaza out of her mind. Somehow she felt her life was entwined with that sandy stretch of Mediterranean seacoast, its turbulent history, and its displaced people.

8

Furlough

"Home Assignment"

What excitement! Mavis surprised her family by arriving forty-five minutes early at the Shreveport Airport on the Ides of March, 1968. Everyone was there—the Lewises, the Odens, the Normans, and the Wylies. *My, how the children have grown*, thought Mavis, and they were all smiles for their "Ankle Bill." Mavis was so happy she didn't even realize that she hadn't slept in twenty-four hours! She could hardly believe she was back with the familiar faces, sights, and smells of Louisiana. It was 1:00 A.M. before she could finally go to sleep because of "jet lag."

The word "furlough" is a misnomer for most missionaries, especially those who are Southern Baptist. The old military term that used to mean "vacation leave" hardly applies to the modern reality. It is often almost impossible to squeeze a vacation into a furlough, as Mavis soon discovered. She barely slept a few hours before she awoke and began sorting slides for the many presentations ahead of her in the churches and other speaking engagements. Mavis was still in a bit of a daze as she attended services that Sunday at the Social Springs Baptist Church where the Women's Missionary Union had formed a "Mavis Pate Circle" as had other churches in Louisiana, Texas, and Mississippi.

Her calendar filled immediately. Before she knew it, every Sunday and most Wednesday evenings were scheduled by churches to hear a report on her work overseas. In addition, there were camps, conferences, and conventions to attend, as well as required medical exams. Furlough quickly became "home assignment."

Mavis enjoyed furlough with a relish, especially eating barbecued venison during a snowstorm in Minden (Louisiana) at Genie and Van Norman's home. She craved cornflakes, lettuce and salads, new potatoes and onions, bell peppers, milk, and the gravy only her mother could make. These were the "favorite things" she had missed in Pakistan. Mavis was unconscious of the austerity to which she had accustomed herself to overseas, as Genie observed:[1]

She always wanted to help with chores when she was in our home, so I often told her to set the table with the dishes and silver. On one occasion, she had set only a salad fork for each person. Van, on arriving at the table, and having no knowledge of who the "helper" was, commented that a child must have set the table because there were no regular-sized forks or other silver. Another time, with hamburgers for the meal, she used paper napkins in setting the table. She tore each napkin into fourths—a holdover from a scarcity of paper products while in East Pakistan.

Mavis's Middle Eastern mentality did come in handy at least once. She bargained with the local car dealer on a 1966 Mustang and got it for $1,700. The car averaged 19.4 miles per gallon when using the air conditioning during the stifling summer.

She set out in the Mustang for Tyler, Texas, for a joyful reunion with Pastor Shamburger at First Baptist Church, where another "Mavis Pate Circle" had been established. Then she zipped across Louisiana to Columbus, Mississippi, to speak at Calvary Baptist and First Baptist churches—all this before returning to Shreveport for a full round of medical and dental exams. Such a whirlwind schedule set the pace for Mavis on furlough. She settled down, only briefly, during scheduled conferences and conventions.

Carville

The Spanish Governor Miro (1785-92) had established a hospital for leprosy patients (Hansen's disease) in New Orleans which led to the establishment of a state leprosarium at Carville in 1894. The federal government took over Carville in 1921. The majority of leprosy cases in the U.S.A. occur in the Gulf coast regions of Florida, Louisiana, and Texas due to the damp, hot climate. About 275 leprosy cases are hospitalized in the federal Public Health Service Hospital at Carville.[2]

Mavis had talked in the past about being from Louisiana and never having been to Carville. Leprosy was and is a major illness in Southeast Asia, and she was compelled to have special training in this area. Now she finally found the opportunity to attend a week-long leprosy seminar at Carville on April 18-24, 1968. The week updated her skills in treating those who suffered from this dreaded disease. She also needed the times of reflection during vespers at the lake and fellowship with Rev. Oscar Harris and his wife, Juanita, who ministered to the spiritual needs of the patients. She left Carville determined to take life a little easier, but her determination was short-lived.

Back in Ringgold, she spent the next few days sewing and writing numerous letters to all her friends overseas. After attending Memorial Day services at Social Springs church, she enjoyed an overnight visit with Johnie Hoyt Oden, her stepbrother, and his wife Carolyn in Waskom, Texas. Mavis had prayed for them and their children many times during her absence. She didn't forget their financial and moral support during the difficult times before appointment. One's family takes on a profound meaning during an overseas absence. She experienced Jesus' promise in Matthew 19:29 that, "every one who has left houses or brothers or sisters or father or mother or children or lands, for my name's sake, will receive a hundredfold, and inherit eternal life." At the same time, it was thrilling to renew ties with her stateside family. But she was hardly settled into being "at home" before she was off again.

Houston

Attending a furloughing missionary conference and the Southern Baptist Convention is a major treat for a missionary on home leave. Mavis was excited that the convention was in Houston, and she could make it in her Mustang. The furloughing conference was at Houston

Baptist College, May 30-June 2, 1968. On arrival, she found, to her delight, that missionary Violett Popp from Lebanon was one of her suite mates. Rogers M. Smith, director of the conference, asked Mavis to give a devotional thought the next morning on "Furlough Reckoning." Then, Dr. Baker James Cauthen inspired her as he preached Sunday evening on "Why call ye Me, Lord, Lord, and do not what I say?"

Mavis felt as though she should walk the aisle to recommit her life to world missions, as she heard more messages at the Woman's Missionary Union conference. The pinnacle of the Convention came on Thursday evening during the presentation on the Convention theme of "Good News for the Nations":[3]

Ronald C. Hill (Thailand), Santiago Canclini (Argentina), Julian C. Bridges (Mexico), Joseph A. Adegbite (Nigeria), and John A. Roper (Jordan) spoke of good news through evangelism and church development through hospitals and medical care. Emphasis was also put on good news through publication work and benevolent ministries. Secretary Cauthen addressed the Convention on good news through support for foreign missionaries. He challenged the Convention messengers to a worthy response to the needs of the world for the good news of Christ.

The high point of the Convention came as Evangelist Billy Graham preached from Titus 2:11-15 on "The Second Coming of Christ." Mavis left weary but affirmed. She was part of a larger family of Christ who, despite their weaknesses, had the world on their heart.

Zackey

The tall Johnson grass thrived despite the sultry heat as Mavis drove over to the post office to pick up her mail in Ringgold. There she met Zackey Meachum, widower and former chairman of deacons. Zackey hoped that Mavis would stay home long enough for them to get acquainted. He learned about Mavis through church publications after she became a missionary. When she finally agreed, he began to visit at her house. Most of their dates were in her parlor, after she cooked thick grilled steaks. Occasionally, they went out to the pizza place.

It was not easy for them to meet for church since she spoke in a different place nearly every Sunday. Mavis shared with Zackey her feelings about the Lord. Basically, she explained, "I was a worldly person until I was converted. You don't know the change that came into my life." He admired her commitment, especially when he observed her friends offering her cigarettes and beer. They said, "Are you sure you've really changed?" She responded, "Yes," and refused. One night she kissed him good-night. He was amused when, on their next date, the first thing she said was, "If you thought I didn't act dedicated to my commitment last night, I'm sorry!"

Their growing friendship placed both Mavis and Zackey in a dilemma. It grew to the point of marriage, it would mean a radical departure from Mavis's commitment to missions. Already her constant absence formeetings and conferences placed a strain on the relationship. When the subject of marriage finally came up, Mavis indicated that she might like to get married and have a family of her own. "If we don't get married I'll be up for reassignment and won't be back in the United States again," she sighed, little realizing the prophetic impact of her words. Zackey cooled the relationship to test her resolve. Mavis was disappointed when they broke up. He later married a pretty former num whom he met on a Mediterranean cruise not far from Gaza![4]

For a while Mavis didn't contact the Foreign Mission Board. Finally on December 17, 1968, she called Dr. J. D. Hughey, area director for Europe and the Middle East and confirmed her decision in the following letter:

Thank you for keeping me so well informed in regards to the proceedings related to the Pakistan hospital project. I truly am eager to begin to make definite plans for the year ahead. I am writing this letter to restate my thoughts as shared in our telephone conversations of this date.

In case the Pakistan hospital project does not develop by January, 1969, I feel led to pursue the following course of action, believing that God will open or close doors along the way to direct my path.

1st—I shall request a transfer to India and shall apply for an entrance visa as soon as I can obtain a new passport.

2nd—If it appears necessary in order to obtain the visa, or if it is deemed necessary by Board personnel staff, I will consider seeking a Master's Degree in Nursing Administration. I realize this would necessitate a leave of absence from the Board.

3rd—If India appears as a closed door to me then I shall request transfer to a place where English is the main language—probably Gaza or Rhodesia.

I'm indeed grateful to you for your understanding thoughtfulness during this time of my seeking God's will and direction.

"Love in Action"

Furlough was not all heartache for Mavis. She rejoiced to see forty-nine young people make commitments to Christ at a Girl's Auxiliary Camp at Tall Timbers near Alexandria, Louisiana (June, 1968). There was also a happy reunion with Dr. Rebekah Naylor while attending a summer session at Southwestern Baptist Theological Seminary. Returning to Southwestern renewed Mavis's prayer life and deepened her resolve for the future.

Back in Minden, Louisiana, Mavis accepted the invitation of Dr. Ronald Prince to speak before the First Baptist Church. She took as her theme, "Love in Action in Pakistan." This was her theme as she attended Foreign Missions Week at Glorieta, and as she participated in World Missions Conferences in Marshfield and Houston, Missouri, in November.

Mavis left no stone unturned in her determination to cover the United States during furlough. She spent the rest of the fall visiting the Loftlands and Howards who were furloughing in Owensboro, Kentucky. The little Mustang took her to Ridgecrest, North Carolina, and to Chattanooga, Tennessee. It made it all the way back through Arkansas in late November, in time to help Van Norman fill a pew on a Friday evening for a revival in Minden. Both she and the Mustang finally gasped to a stop when she contracted laryngitis after Christmas and took a much needed rest!

A letter arrived from Dr. Hughey on January 22, 1969, approving Mavis's return to Pakistan. The political situation continued to be uncertain, and February found Mavis "earnest in prayer for the missionaries. But God gave me assurance." Social Springs church celebrated a "Mavis Pate Day" on February 16 and gave her a love gift of money. Pastor Kennedy later remarked, "Mavis had a dramatic spiritual impact on our church while she was here on furlough. We could not have her in our midst and remain the same." Mavis spoke almost 100 times in different churches and meetings during her year of furlough. In all, she received $2,003.07 in furlough love offerings, honoraria, and expenses from the churches in which she spoke, testifying to their generosity and her popularity. Only one time did Mavis forget to feed the little Mustang, as Genie recalled:

She had absolutely *no* personal fear and trusted implicitly in God's care over her. We who loved and cared for her cautioned her often about the many travels in her old used car . . . Once while returning from a speaking engagement, she ran out of gas on an Interstate Highway several miles from the nearest exit . . . She then got out and started the walk to the nearest help. Soon a man stopped for she was walking along this major highway *in a sari*, which she had worn for the speech earlier. Whether curious or caring, he took her to a service station, obtained the necessary fuel, and engaged in conversation with another customer who was traveling the direction from which she had come. After much insistence, the "new" Samaritan was allowed to return her to her car and she was on her way. Our usual "You really *should* be more careful" was met with, "Who would harm a missionary, in her 40's, walking on an Interstate Highway . . . wearing a sari?"

The furlough year was blessed, but it had to end. All the pizza, crawfish etufe, and quail dinners were soon memories, along with the adulation of family and multitudes of friends in the churches. Returning to the field was like "setting one's hands to the plow and not looking back." It was not easy, but it had to be done for the Kingdom's sake. On March 1, 1969, at Shreveport Airport, Mavis's mother and stepfather, Gwen, Pam, and Genie were there to see her off. The Loftlands met her for a short stopover in Dallas. Then she was off to Seattle for the flight over the Pacific . . . and toward the future!

9

East Pakistan: Part IV

Reorientation

Readjusting to life in East Pakistan was easier than Mavis expected. Now with furlough completed she began to catch the feeling of the land, the people, and the mission:

In addition to getting a nest made, be it temporary or permanent, I have been trying to feel the pulse of the country, the mission, and myself. I think one is as difficult to determine as the other since all are so intermingled and interdependent. There is so much to do so many places, just to know my specific place is all I can ask. Pray with me for that. Pray with me that the happiness and the peace be increased in the world by means of God's love and presence and that I will be a part of helping make this so.[1]

Peace evaded the land. Bengali-speaking East Pakistanis chafed under the pressures of the ruling Urdu-speaking leaders of West Pakistan. The Urdus felt that they followed a purer form of Islam than that of their Bengali cousins. They suspected India of supporting a growing independence movement in the country. Unknown to Mavis, the tension influenced the government decision not to grant permission to build the new hospital. Officials were more than willing to sacrifice this needed Christian institution to pacify fanatic Islamic leadership.

Martial Law

Tensions mounted in the country as the discontented Bengalis led a torchlight parade one Sunday evening. The next morning business was at a standstill outside Mavis's window. She could hear the marching and chanting of protesters. Later three theaters were burned. Returning from a trip to Faridpur on March 27, 1969, she found that the government had imposed martial law on the country: "The latter was noted only a military compound across the street in the small hours of the morning prior to the day it went into effect, then a peaceful calm and relaxing of tensions as everyone went about their business."[2]

The negative side of martial law restricted the holding of meetings. Mavis thought about opening immunization clinics and beginning classes on planned parenthood. The new situation led her to think of reasons why she should stay in the country and also reasons why she should leave. *Is it a waste of stewardship of talents to go into this work?* she asked herself as she pondered the pros and cons.

She assured the folks back home that "we see and are involved in very little, so do not be concerned about us. We learn most of the news and happenings from the same source you do!"[3] Enduring the oppressive heat, remaking old friends, witnessing to a few new ones, and directing rickshaws through mazes of downtown traffic kept her too busy to be concerned about the political situation. The mission wisely placed the burden of the Guest House on her again! This satisfied to an extent her gregarious nature. But it required more than this to convince her that East Pakistan should remain her home for the moment.

Tornado

It took a storm to firm up Mavis's resolve to remain in the country, as she related on April 14, 1969:

Texas dust storms should have had me prepared for this day's weather. Dust, rain, and hail in spots, wind strong enough to send tin sailing through the air, and more dust. The wind is still blowing quite strongly, the electricity has been off for several hours now. My light is a candle and my "Houston" kerosene lantern . . . It's quite obvious that at the time I wrote the beginning of this letter that I did not know the extent of the storm clouds and the strong wind! The tornado hit the other side of town about the time I was on the way from the Guest House that afternoon. I saw black clouds but did not hear how bad it was until the next day. When I did, I went over to the Holy Family Hospital to help out. I spent most of the day cleaning and dressing cuts. Records showed that they treated 228 patients there. Voice of America said 1000 were dead and 4000 injured![4]

The storm, the affirmation of friends, and being able to serve in the hospital in a time of need, were for Mavis the Lord's way of saying, "Stay for now." *It's good to have the decision made. The drastic need, to be here at such a time and to be able to help in the storm, seemed a benediction to the decision;* she thought. She shared with family and Dr. J. D. Hughey in the form of a Japanese Haiku, a type of poem with seventeen syllables:

> After the long night—
> Pakistan will be my home
> He leads—rays of light.

"I am convinced that God has put me back in this place at this time for His purpose and plan though I still 'see through the glass darkly.' " New activities momentarily shed some light, along with frustrations, on her path.[5]

Social-Service Center

Children swarmed everywhere, as Mavis and the summer missionary tried to maintain control in the sweltering heat. Sixty-five showed up for the children's recreation time at the new social service center in Mirpur. *Some contrast to the few who showed up to get immunized!* she mused. One of the youngsters suggested she might have more participation, "if you offered them something nicer than shots!"

Despite Mavis's spirit, she still found it difficult to get out and invite people to come in, but the experience proved a breakthrough for her:

All the week prior to a "Get-Acquainted Tea" for the ladies of Mirpur I spent in going house-to-house introducing myself, telling of the work of the center and inviting the ladies to the tea. At first I quaked in my

boots but went anyway. It was a delightful experience and I was received very graciously every place that I went. The results were gratifying in that approximately forty women and thirty to thirty-five children came to the tea. They were women from all levels of society
including a doctor and a doctor's wife.

With this positive experience behind her she even got up enough
nerve to have a snake-charmer brought in to "demonstrate his skill
with his captives. My sincere wish is that they remain his captives and
stay in the basket!"[6]

The presence of summer missionaries highlighted the season for
Mavis. These vibrant volunteers, from Baptist Student Unions in the
United States, lifted her spirits. "It renews one's faith in the younger
generation to see their wholesome attitudes and lives." Also, the professional and personal companionship of Benita Brothers, public-
health nurse on short-term volunteer service, made the busy summer
worthwhile. "She was here just long enough for me to realize how nice
it was to have someone to share work and worries and meals with."
Together they performed several "Good News" musical concerts for
the missionaries and the Bengalis who remarked, "Did you say that
you would be doing something like this every week from now on?"

Mirpur set the pace for the opening of another smaller center in
Tongi on August 28, 1969. Mavis hoped to assist in follow-up of tu-
berculosis patients from a government clinic in Tongi. In September
she treated more than 140 patients in a week-long clinic in Faridpur,
assisted by the ladies of the church. When she wrote home she shared
her frustration and faith:

I have discovered that my greatest need of the moment is a computer
for differential diagnosis and treatment of tropical diseases, of all the
diseases found in Pakistan. I never realized how much alike everybody's symptoms sound, nor how much I did not know about so many
things. My one consolation is that God doubtless honors honest effort
and honest mistakes. He can use any and all to glorify His name.[7]

Mavis enjoyed being involved in this work, but she desired more to see local leadership involved. As this slowly developed, she once again began to search for the way that God would lead her.

About this time she received a letter from Ava Nell McWhorter in Gaza. Their OR nurse had returned to the States for her wedding. Would Mavis be willing to transfer to Gaza to fill this need? Mavis replied that she had just set up the public-health work and needed more time. She and Ava Nell covenanted to pray about it. They figured out the time difference and agreed to pray at 10:00 A.M. each morning.

Fishing Boats

Pakistani fishing boats paralleled Mavis's life at that time. As she described the boats, "It is a one-man boat. It is shaped like the bottom half of a washpot (anyone know what a washpot is?), made out of clay baked to a hard finish. One sits in it and whirls and paddles along."[8] The world was a whirl of activity around her. Somehow, there was forward motion, but the direction was not yet certain.

An enjoyable part of the whirl was being "Ankle Bill" to Tom and Gloria Thurman for the birth of David Olive Thurman in October 1969. His big brother Philip seemed as anxious to be on hand for the event as Mavis, despite his suffering a sore throat and cold. This event almost eclipsed the parade of the astronauts through Dacca a few days later.

The political whirl increased; violence broke out in the city as citizens protested over having to vote with ballots in Urdu, as well as Bengali. The subsequent curfew quieted the city to a deafening silence. During this time it gave her incentive to hire a "compounder" or druggist to supervise the supply of low-cost drugs for the centers. She discovered that the local people willingly responded to the need if she innovated and shared responsibility. The girls at Mirpur center rose to the challenge by adapting their own version of "Good Deed Dottie," a children's game, as they went home chanting "Bhalo Khajer Kholi," "Kholi" being the Bengali equivalent of "Dottie."

The Pakistani whirl transported Mavis on a trip to the East Pakistan Tea Gardens in Sylhet. Then she traveled on five ferries and over 137 miles to visit Dr. Fidelia Gilbert in Bogra before attending the mission retreat in Kaptai. The whirl did not take her eyes off of one important goal—Bengali studies! Tucked in between all the activities she continued to upgrade her language capability. On December of 1969 she successfully completed a two-and-a-half hour written exam and a one-hour oral test in Bengali. The whirl of the Pakistani boat began to slow down. A Macedonian call brought it to a stop on the shores of the Middle East.

Transfer

Throughout all the activities, the question kept running through Mavis's mind, *Is this the best stewardship of my talents? The Lord knows that the operating room is my first love!* Jim McKinley shared Mavis's dilemma: "Mavis seemed always to want the will of God above everything else. She visited Feni, where the hospital would have been built while my family lived there. Night after night she and I talked long after Betty and our children had gone to bed. She would often say, 'But I want to do what God wants.' "[9] In a letter to her family, she shared fresh insight into what she thought God wanted:

These past nine months in Pakistan have been my busiest ones here, and they have been my happiest ones. Just goes to prove a principle of life that we all know, doesn't it? Keep busy and keep out of trouble and keep happier. It's a challenge to see if I could find the handle of something different and lift the lid enough to know something of what is inside a different field of endeavor . . . BUT, when I heard that the Gaza Hospital was losing their operating-room nurse to the field of matrimony I got all goose-pimply thinking, *Maybe, just maybe the Lord will open the way to that for me . . . to operating room nursing and to matrimony. Ha! But the operating room I was thinking about for a beginning!*

Several made trips through Dacca with news from Richmond and Gaza, to the extent that I was aware that a request for such a transfer at this time would be favorably received and that an invitation would be forthcoming. So, as of January 1, 1970 I officially requested a transfer to Gaza Hospital.

The encouragement of her friends helped Mavis make the decision to transfer. Tom and Gloria Thurman, Jim McKinley, and Bill Marshall, then the field representative for the Foreign Mission Board in the Middle East, spent long and agonizing hours with her. Jim confirmed the "family decision" that affirmed Mavis's choice:

When it became a reality that the Government of East Pakistan would not permit the building of the hospitals, some of us had doubts about Mavis remaining. She had great talents in nursing. While she may have felt relatively good about working in a little social-service center, we knew she could be doing much more than that. I talked to her about this and she seemed to be relieved. So, finally when the decision was made to leave East Pakistan, it had not been made by her alone. Her colleagues tried to be an encouragement so she would feel free to go to a place where her gifts could be put to greater use. When she left, she knew she had the blessings of her colleagues.[10]

Mavis spiritually stepped out of the whirling Pakistani boat and set sail on the ship of faith headed toward the Holy Land. It was not an easy decision. She had become firmly attached to the land and had finally become conversant with the language. People responded to her amiable nature. Some began to mimic her efficiency and initiative. But as she shared in a letter to Dr. Hughey, "I have been led to the conviction that according to the gift of ability the Spirit has given me, I can serve the body better in the Gaza hospital."[11]

She voiced two major concerns in leaving. First, she longed to see the success of the social-service centers she helped to start. They were still like tender plants that needed much care and nurture to stand on their own. These she trusted to the Lord and the faithfulness of national and missionary partners she left behind. The other major concern was how her mother would react to the news of the transfer. "Help convince Mother that I am in no more danger there. Try to help her see it objectively. I do feel anxious to get back into a hospital," she pleaded with her sister Gwen.[12] The news coming from the Middle East did not give much assurance to Mattie!

Farewells

Selling all her belongings didn't come easy to Mavis. "It's hard to stand by and let people plow through the meager belongings one has managed to collect over the years." As she cleaned her closets she stopped and bid each piece a little farewell. She was allowed 100 pounds of unaccompanied baggage by air in addition to the usual forty-four pounds. She sent a few boxes of books and a barrel via Cyprus. The rest had to be sold to missionary and Bengali friends. The weariness of packing and finishing up last-minute business made her want to stay " 'til Kingdom come!" She distributed leftover books and Bibles to the reading rooms and beggar friends as she made her last rounds in Dacca.

Each farewell tugged on her heart. "Achievement Day" at the Mirpur Center overwhelmed her as the children placed three leis around her neck, so high she could hardly see over them. "Farewells are getting more and more difficult to say. Whatever will I do by another furlough time? If God requires it He must give the strength!" Strength did come through the inspiration of worship. "Tonight we sang 'We will follow the steps of Jesus, where'er they go.' " The thought came to me, *What better way than to go start a journey where He began His, in Bethlehem?* In response to a message from Dr. Boyd in Louisiana Mavis replied, "Tell him I feel like I am headed back where I belong!"[13] On February 13, 1970, while nursing a case of laryngitis, Mavis flew to Karachi en route to Beirut and Nicosia, to the place she firmly believed she belonged—Gaza.

10
Gaza: Part I

1970

The noise of the marketplace across from the Gaza Baptist Hospital compound awoke Mavis at 5 A.M. She shook her head and tried orienting herself for a moment. Then she began to recollect the events of the last few days—first, the delay at the Beirut airport when security discovered her Israeli visa in her passport and refused to permit her to leave the passenger lounge . . . then, the night in Nicosia when the hotel was full and the manager invited her home to spend the night with him and his wife. The trips to Famagusta and Kyrenia with the Bill Marshalls flicked through her mind, almost blurring with her arrival at the Ben-Gurion Airport near Tel Aviv. Ava Nell McWhorter and others from the Gaza Baptist Hospital staff greeted her. In Gaza, they combined greetings and farewells in a party for her and nurse Pat Haile who was returning to the States. Then she took a whirlwind trip to Baptist Village, the airport, Jerusalem, and Bethlehem to check on freight and an apartment for language study. Now, back in Gaza for the weekend, a cold splash of water on the face shocked Mavis into reality. *Today, I'll take a look at the operating room!* she thought, as she braced herself against the February chill.

Mavis's reputation as a strict operating-room nurse had preceded her to Gaza. Ava Nell remembered Mavis's professionalism from earlier days in Louisiana:[1]

We first met in Shreveport in 1952 where she was operating room supervisor at Charity Hospital. I was instructor for the Northwestern

School of Nursing. She was about five years older than I. Our students did their clinical work at Charity. The students were awed and frightened of her. She was a stickler, all business in the operating room. The interns toed the mark! She demanded that others do what they were supposed to do. But when you got to know her you realized she was a warm person. It was amazing how rigid she was at work, but in everyday life she was really a fun-loving person.

The person most likely to be affected by Mavis's professional attitude was Jane Yates. Journeyman nurse from Washington state, Jane supervised the operating room, in the interim, until Mavis finished a short course in Arabic. Mavis was already a "giant" in Jane's eyes because of her reputation from the *Ship Hope:*[2]

I was brand new. She was a seasoned nurse. Though I had a B.S. in Nursing from Baylor, Gaza was on-the-job training for me. I was self-conscious that Mavis would be critical. I was not an OR nurse, though I knew the standard techniques.

She went to Bethlehem to study language and would come home on the weekends. She did not come snooping around. She never did interfere or make any statement about what was or was not being done. That was rather big of her. There would have been plenty for her to say had she chosen to. She was not condescending. She went about her business of language study. She was not one who needed her ego stroked a lot. She did a lot of things that were acknowledged.

After Jane showed Mavis around the operating room, Mavis's only reflection in a letter home was, "much, *much* to do there!!"

Political tension punctuated regularly by violence is a constant reality in Gaza. Throughout its long history Gaza has been the trampling ground of numerous conquerors, with Egypt to the south and Syria to the north. Since the war in 1967, it has been the scene of the frustrated struggle of Palestinians against the Israeli Army of Occupation. Mavis felt the tension as she watched Israeli soldiers guarding every street corner and heard the rumble of half-trucks mounted with machine guns on routine patrol. The hospital staff braced for action every time the frustration erupted. A hand grenade would be lobbed at a patrol. More often than not it missed its mark, rolling into a shop or crowded marketplace, and blowing up, maiming and killing the innocent. The second weekend Mavis spent in Gaza in February 1970, thirteen persons were wounded in such a bombing. Two days later she witnessed a small explosion only a half-block away. In a similar incident the windshield of hospital chaplain Ed Nicholas's car was blown out. The foreign staff was not complacent, but they always thought *they* would be excepted from such violence.

Bethlehem—Arabic Studies

Don't know whether I'm going to find time to settle down and begin language study or not. You know, I may be completely ruined as a 7 to 3 regular after these past seven years, thought Mavis as she faced Arabic studies and returned to hospital life. Visiting the holy places with new missionary friends eased the transition.[4]

Receiving shipments, arranging visas, and returning social obligations to those who had welcomed her to Gaza consumed the first few weeks. Soon, she moved up to Bethlehem to begin Arabic studies. Mavis tired of "playing like a tourist" and was "anxious to get on with this study, learn this Arabic in short order, and get back down to Gaza to get that apartment set up and get to work!"

Her partners in Arabic studies were Jarrell and Shirley Peach from Missouri. Jarrell was a physiotherapist appointed by Southern Baptists to set up a physiotherapy clinic at the Gaza Hospital. Mr. Jalil Irani, a veteran language teacher and Arabic scholar, taught them. His father had converted from the Bahai faith. The founders of the Bahai religion had been exiled from Iran to Haifa and Acre during the British Mandate. With five lessons behind her Mavis commented, "It's just as humbling as Bengali—Wow!"

Mavis immediately took to the Peach children, Cari Lynn, age 5, and Jay, 3, whom she considered "dolls." She and the Peaches shared a VW station wagon assigned to them by the Gaza Mission. They usually made the trip to Gaza every weekend. Mavis found them to be compatible companions, particularly when they shared her embarrassment as she made mistakes in Arabic class.

The Easter holidays arrived and afforded a hiatus from language study. Mavis followed the Good Friday procession from the Mount of Olives to Pilate's courtyard on the Via Dolorosa. Then she enjoyed a picnic at Shepherd's field near Bethlehem. An Easter sunrise service at the Garden Tomb and a worship service at the Baptist Church with Bill Marshall preaching made it a special day. A few days later she attended the Israel Mission annual meeting, which met as a separate organization from the Gaza Mission. A week later she was surprised to find the members of the Greek Orthodox Church celebrating Easter!

"Language study is a tedious grind. I'm glad it will only be for a four-month period. When the end is in sight it is easier to 'get the medicine down!' " fretted Mavis in a letter home. Already behind with her studies, Mavis chafed from having to move from the Arab Women's Union Club near Mr. Irani's home to Bet Jala, a neighboring town. This meant about a half-hour walk to language study. But she enjoyed the spacious quarters and the privacy. The Arab-style bathrooms fascinated her:[5]

The Arabic bathroom features a commode built into the floor with a place for the feet at each side. It flushes with an overhead tank called a "Niagara." Some in older homes flush by pouring water into them. There is a water faucet close to it so they don't have to use the little water pitcher as people do in Pakistan. The other bath has a regular hand-washing sink, a bathtub, and regular commode, a hot-water heater and, as little Jay Peach (age 3) said, a "nice little tub for babies." Only it sits just to the side of the commode, is about the same height, and has a similar rim without a seat. It has a similar stopper in the bottom and a fountainlike spout. That is the ultramodern type of Eastern toilet tissue. The hot-water heater looks much the same as a gas or electric tank, but it has a "fire-box" underneath it. I could not have hot water for the first couple of days until I went out and bought some wood. Everything would have been fine if the wood had not been green. I need some good kindling. All the principles of "laying a good fire" are coming back to me. I fire up the "geyser" and have a good bath every other night.

Mavis had the ability to see the humorous in the mundane. This kept her going through Arabic studies. She found herself progressing faster in Arabic than she had in Bengali, due probably to the fact that she was more motivated. The weekly fellowship with the Gaza missionaries and occasional trips to Baptist Village in Israel encouraged her. She received particular pleasure from getting acquainted with her Arab neighbors:

I'm enjoying being in the apartment more than in the Club. The landladies (best I can tell there are three spinster sisters, their brother and his wife and five children who live upstairs) and the landlord are very gracious. One of the sisters is a schoolteacher and helps me with my Arabic. She makes me read aloud, and that is something I cannot get myself to sit down and do.

Yesterday while I was out for a walk with the teacher, the one who keeps a garden (in it are apricot trees, olive trees, akadinia trees, mulberry trees, grapevines, almond trees, onions, garlic, cabbage, roses, sweet peas, snapdragons, and a few things I have probably missed!) fell and broke her collarbone. They came for the sister so I went along. Needless to say I was a little disappointed when they went to call an old, feeble lady (a medicine lady I guess) who rubbed it well with salve, placed a splint about the size of a tongue depressor over the broken bone, put an Ace bandage around her shoulders and shook her head sadly. I must admit the bandage was applied somewhat on the order of a figure-eight bandage but certainly did not pull the bone into place. I heard that she was back this morning and said everything was all right.

Mavis found the Arab people more friendly and outgoing than the Pakistanis. She marveled at the cleaning lady who insisted that Mavis have one of her bananas. "In Pakistan they would insist on having one of mine!" she mused. Especially did she enjoy the Arabic food and hospitality:[6]

Just as soon as my eyes were open, the upstairs neighbors invited me out to pick apricots off the tree and eat. They served Arabic or Turkish coffee. That is the expresso kind, very thick, black, and sweet. Then they gave me a fresh baked loaf of Arabic bread. It reminds me of

Grandma Johnson's "big biscuits" or "hoe cakes." It has a little yeast, is made the night before, let rise, and cooked over hot coals the next morning . . .

The next day I was invited by the secretary of the Club where I lived in Bethlehem to her home for lunch. They had a small banquet including 'qusa ma'shi' (stuffed squash with rice and meat), broiled chicken, 'warak dewali' (rice and meat wrapped in young tender grape leaves and steamed), 'sfiha' (small half-moon pies with meat inside), salad of tomatoes and cucumber (much like ours), a rice dish much like fried rice, but each person dips into the same dish, and beer. The family is Catholic and they were astonished that I did not choose to drink beer. For dessert they had a large sampling of the lovely summer fruits, mulberry, apricots, plums, and watermelons. Then you go to the living room and have coffee.

Do you think my day ended there? The upstairs neighbors invited me for supper to eat the very popular national dish, "mansef." That is a delicious rice dish made very rich with yogurt, nuts, and served with mutton that is pan roasted with spices, or boiled. Tasty and rich!

You will not be surprised that I and all the Arab women are big! This P.M. I went to visit a lady with my landlady. We had two glasses of lemonade, jello, ice cream, bananas and green, green grapes. Now I have sunflower seed and am expected at friends for dessert in ten minutes!

Language study was not all eating and feasting for Mavis. As she absorbed the language she found more opportunities to share her faith with others. This made the humiliation of having to start again as a "first-grader" worthwhile:

So far my main opportunities to witness have been to Muslim women—and, Oh, does Christianity have much to offer them. The Muslim here is much more liberal than in Pakistan but still bound and tied by "laws" and rituals and dogmatism. Though it is probably hard to realize, I have little contact with Jewish people. About the only ones I talk with are the soldiers at road checkpoints or in government offices. The girl who cleans this big apartment for me is a high school girl, 15, and a Muslim. I asked her to come by just for a visit when she was not going to work. She did Saturday morning and got me out of bed! Thank goodness she did not let that run her off. We had a good time trying to talk Arabic. Not nearly all I need but God can use some poor efforts, by human standards. Fatima took a leaflet about the correspondence course. Maybe she will have some time while out of school and will use it. Her father is dead. She has three brothers and her mother. Let's pray together for her.

Made another friend when in Gaza last time. She had fallen from a moving car. She was about 16 years old. She grasped my hand and almost pleaded that I stop and talk with her after the movie was over on the women's ward. See, it is not hard to find opportunity to talk to people about Christ. She just wanted to talk to the "foreign lady" but we talked a little about everything, laughed together, and learned more about each other. She is engaged to be married (arranged by father); her husband will not wait until she finishes high school in one year. Her father has three wives (no, she does not like co-wives). She does not want to get married, but her father will beat her if she does not.

Being able to share in the heartaches of others gave Mavis an incentive to study Arabic. The Arabs practically worship their language. They admire anyone who is willing to study it. The four months of Arabic studies in Bethlehem passed before Mavis realized it. She attended her last lesson with Mr. Irani in June of 1970 and recorded the Model Prayer in Arabic. Fatima came in the next day to help her clean house. She ate another fabulous Arab breakfast with the neighbors and packed. She would not forget them.

OR Duty

The Gaza Baptist Hospital compound buzzed with activity. Mavis's day began with her quiet time at 5:00 A.M. Then she prepared herself for an 8:30 to 3:00 P.M. shift in the OR. In the summer, numerous volunteers came through, and she usually found herself volunteering to take them on tours of the Holy Land. This offered her a discreet way to complete her own "orientation" to the land. The numerous social functions in the evening for the new arrivals or those leaving made it as difficult for Mavis to control her food intake as it had been in Bethlehem!

The first order of the day was to debrief with Jane Yates and "drain her brain" about the operating-room procedures. Mavis feared that her relationship to the staff and fellow missionaries would suffer if she pressed too hard on reforms. She wrote home:[7]

I ask the prayers of all of you that I go about my work here in the way God would have it. There is much to do in the OR, but I do not want to rush into it too quickly or be discouraged with the fact that I may not be able to do all the things I would like to do. You know how important going about things in the right way is when there is as much "togetherness" as there is in this situation.

"Togetherness" was forced on Mavis a little before she was prepared for it. The second day she had charge of the OR, Ava Nell had to go somewhere. She told Mavis, "You are on your own!" An Arab Christian nurse and a third-year Muslim nursing student got into an argument. They pushed and slapped. Mavis wanted to call Ava Nell or Dr. Roy McGlamery, director of the hospital, for help, but they were not to be found. In desperation she locked the Christian in her office and sent the Muslim home for the day. Later, Ava Nell told her that as long as she had a lock on her office that was the best thing to do!

The Gaza Baptist Hospital had been taken over from the Church Missionary Society of the Episcopal Church in 1954. The United Nations referred most of its surgery cases to the hospital. This kept the operating room busy with three or four major cases every other day and lots of "little stuff," as Mavis put it. Some days this meant up to twenty cases. The lack of preparation of supplies, and the alternating schedule frustrated Mavis. Added to this she began Arabic studies again. Then came some disturbing news from the Thurmans in East Pakistan:[8]

I must share this bad news with all of you to ask specially that you add your prayer to mine. Before I left Pakistan, Gloria showed me a spot on her instep that grossly appeared to be ringworm. It was very sensitive in the center. Gloria saw her obstetrician, and she thought likewise. The medication given did not clear it. In several weeks the center of the lesion became insensitive. When Gloria was taking David to the skin specialist about a fungus, she said, "I'll ask about this too." The spot was diagnosed as Hansen's Disease, that is, leprosy. You can imagine everyone's shock and dismay. However, God is good! This type which gives this appearance is the mildest type and the easiest to cure. The doctor put her on sulfone treatment, and I have learned that if things go well he will not recommend going home.

You should have seen the letter Gloria wrote telling me about this. As always, her faith and strength shone through giving inspiration to others rather than giving any indication of needing strength from others. But even at that we know how much love and prayers and encouragement she needs. Oh, how I wish I could be with her to help at such a time!

Gloria's illness and even a little "nit" like finding a mango in the market brought back nostalgia for Pakistan. "I was in Pakistan long enough that I get homesick for some of the things from there now. Mostly for friends, mango, papaya, and good bananas, rice, and curry!"

The OR schedule kept Mavis so busy she nearly missed seeing Aubrey and Norma Pate, relatives from Louisiana who were on a tour of the Holy Land. They arrived in Gaza on a Thursday which was an operating day. Mavis planned to have lunch with them but did not get out of the OR until 4:30 in the afternoon!

As summer ended and the staff started going on vacation, Mavis inherited the responsibility for central supply. Her nerves began to fray:

Pray with me that my patience will hold out through all this. Is it the age, you think, or the language and cultural barrier? Well, when you put them both together, I seem to come up with moments of "snarling." That ain't good!

Ava Nell vividly remembers one of those moments of "snarling":[9]

"We had only one run-in in our eighteen months together. You really had to communicate with her. I am prone to do things and not let people know. I had asked her to take over central supply and steriliza-tion. She was off for the day. They called me down. Something was wrong with the autoclave. I had Doctor 'Mac' call Tel Aviv to order a new one. The next morning she went into central supply, and the man told her it was broken. She wrote out a purchase order and went to the office and found out it had already been ordered! About an hour later I met her on the balcony and she said, 'If you want me to take care of central service I would appreciate your keeping your nose out of it!' So I said, 'Maybe we ought to talk.' When she said that, I was not really sure what the problem was all about. So we went up to the office and I found out. Then I explained, 'When you are off, I am responsible. If I do something in your area of responsibility, tell me. But don't blast me!' It never happened again."

Revival

A constant stream of visitors from the Foreign Mission Board and medical volunteers lifted Mavis's spirits. There were the Betheas, Dr. J. D. Hughey, Dr. Halbrooks, the Van Landinghams, and Dr. Helen Falls. Dr. Merrill Moore and his wife Patty and children returned from furlough and Dr. John Wikman and wife Barbara, who had been re-placing them, returned to India. But the greatest encouragement came from the 175 Arab children enrolled in Vacation Bible School and a youth revival that followed. George Laty, deacon evangelist from the Nazareth Baptist Church, gave an inspiring challenge to the youth: On Wednesday at the 4:30 service (early because of the curfew) at the time of invitation one person went to the altar to make his decision known, and it seemed that the floodgates were opened. More than twenty young people went forward. One young man stood to say, "I am requesting baptism. Won't some of the rest of you come and stand with me for this purpose?" None stood specifically for baptism, but many made public their stand for Christ.

Being of Greek Orthodox families, most had been baptized as in-fants and their families object very strenuously to their accepting be-liever's baptism. It is considered an insult to their practices.

That was not all. The conference went on, and on Friday afternoon there was another manifestation of the work of the Holy Spirit on the group. Again, many stood and went forward for the call to a decision. Among them was a man from a family here who has been recently married. His wife is now my Arabic teacher. I understand that he is an alcoholic. He made a decision. What a vivid witness that will be if he is strengthened to overcome the alcohol in his life.

The revival continued. Another young man decided to follow the Lord in believer's baptism. He publicly suffered the consequences:[10]

In the face of the talk and the discrimination here, he talked at first about being baptized some place other than Gaza. He finally decided to be baptized here. It was a glorious occasion, and one that glorified the Lord. After the night church service in which he was baptized there was a singspiration which everyone attended. Because it was a big occasion there was a reception with refreshments. During the activities, someone came to the door and asked to see the boy whose name is Immanuel. Immanuel went to the door. Without one word the visitor socked him in the jaw, and he went sprawling on the floor. Someone immediately said, "Stop that man. Don't let him leave through the gate!" But Immanuel came to enough to say, "Please, let him go. It is all right. That was my brother." So the activities continued for some time, and then the boy's father appeared at the door. (None of his family sympathized with his decision or approved of his baptism.) His father was very apologetic for the actions of the other son and invited his newly baptized son to return any time he chose to his home and assured him he was welcome there. No doubt there will still be many obstacles and much difficulty along the way but that in itself was a big victory for him. And his response to the situation was one that glorifies Christ. They say that this boy was quite a ruffian until his recent conversion. Now he is a likable, cheerful, outgoing person, not a polished gentleman, but the same boy who is for Christ now.

Mavis herself opened her heart to spiritual renewal. During a visit to Baptist Village she and Sarah Bivins sat for an hour at the swimming pool and shared about the work of the Holy Spirit. Mavis remarked "I want the fullness of the Holy Spirit!" Sarah concurred. Mavis reflected:[11]

I can hardly believe some of these unbelievable things that are happening in a civilized world, but then we are told that times such as these will be and that Christ is the only solution. It can only make us more positive that His word is true and more assured that He is the answer and that this life is just what we do while waiting for His return and glorious eternal life with Him. Some people must feel awfully hopeless and uncertain without this to lean on.

Nasser

Mavis taught classes in OR nursing and techniques in September with high hopes. But she soon learned the second-year OR students were not up to her standards. She remarked one day to Bertha Jane Marshall, director of nursing, "This is the worst bunch of students I've ever had." "But," replied Bertha Jane, "these are the best students we have!" About two weeks later Mavis told her, "I want to apologize. Your class was really one of the most marvelous I have ever taught." Mavis began to realize the struggle the students were having with English as a second language.

The students were also caught up in the political complications that plagued the Gaza strip. They pinned their hopes on one man to free them from the humiliation of Israeli occupation—Gamal Abdul Nasser. Despite the defeat he suffered at the hands of Israel in 1967, he was still the Arab hero. His picture was on the walls of almost every home. September 29, 1970, the day of his unexpected death, ushered in widespread grief to Gaza:[12]

You cannot imagine the pall that fell over the country the day of Nasser's death. That morning in chapel the girl nurses just sobbed aloud. Though the people were once under the Egyptian rule and fared little better, they look back on it as Utopia and eulogize him as the Beloved of Mohammed now. We are running on a skeleton crew and do things very quietly for these three days.

Mavis assured the folks back home that she kept a low profile outside the hospital compound, particularly since the hijacking and destroying of four airliners in Jordan. Difficulties with the nursing students concerned her more:[13]

After three of the graduate nurses and Mavis's only staff nurse threatened to resign, Mavis began to question her approach:[14]

I am a true example of the type of operating-room supervisor that should not be. I read in a book someplace, do not go in and try to change everything at one time. Take it slow and change only one thing at a time. Well, what is one to do when the Mayo tables are not adequately covered, the linen all has holes in it, the septic case procedure spreads more bacteria than it destroys? The result of the situation is that the days we do not have surgery are busier than the days we do, as I try to get new linens made, have in-service classes, change procedures, and introduce new ones.

Mavis received good news from East Pakistan. Gloria Thurman responded to treatment, and the people in Faridpur missed the "Lady Doctor," as she had come to be called.

Mount of Beatitudes

The wives of the Israel Baptist mission invited the women of the Gaza mission to share in a retreat on the Mount of Beatitudes above the Sea of Galilee in November 1970. Mavis was anxious for a change of pace. She needed the inspiration. With Thanksgiving and the Muslim Eid al Fitr behind, the weather was beginning to cool. Mavis noticed also that there had been no grenade injuries in the last two weeks! As she thought about what to wear and to carry for her share of the refreshments, she cooled a bit to the idea of having to prepare two devotions on the Beatitudes. But the week more than met her expectations:[15]

Whatever this week has been (Advent for one thing) there should be more like it. The trip was marvelous to Tiberias. We stayed on the Mount of Beatitudes above the Sea of Galilee where the Italian Sisters have a chapel and a hostel. They serve meals family style, there are rooms with the scantiest furniture and a bath on the same floor. It is all very comfortable but not luxurious. The retreat was a very relaxed type program and lots of opportunities for laughs.

Mavis visited Eddie Fields and her husband Bob in Jerusalem, where Eddie directed the Jerusalem House Student Center. Then they made a trip to Gaza to visit Mavis. They talked about the fullness of the Holy Spirit. Mavis had read Watchman Nee's book, *Release of the Spirit*.[16] Eddie noted that Mavis was really searching for a constant, day-by-day, moment-by-moment walk in the Spirit. Mavis prayed that night, "I want to know God face to face!"

Shepherd's Field

Christmas in Gaza was unusually cold. The climax of a tremendously heavy year caused Mavis to think back over all that had happened. She remembered with some nostalgia her Pakistani cook who said, "I forgive you for being angry with me." He died three months later. She hoped the Gaza students would be as forgiving. The pace at the hospital had been what she considered "frantic." Christmas was marred in Gaza by the refusal of Greek Orthodox Christians to decorate their homes as a gesture of mourning over the Israeli occupation. She enjoyed welcoming Dr. Jeanne Dickman back from furlough by preparing a curry dinner for her. Together with nurse Anne Dwyer and journeyman Don Roberts they headed for Bethlehem to celebrate a real Christmas.

The program at Shepherd's Field began in the afternoon. Mavis's group fortunately received permits to get almost to the spot by car. Shepherd's Field in the Valley of Boaz lies about two miles below Bethlehem in the modern Arab village of Bet Sahur. After hearing a program in English and Swedish they drove back to the Peaches's home, where Jarrell convalesced from a bout with hepatitis. Later they returned to Shepherd's Field for a worship service led by the Bible Presbyterians and then to the carol singing on Manger Square. "It is marvelous," remarked Mavis, "to be on the spot where it all happened so long ago!" The experience inspired her to pen the following verses:[17]

I want to go to Shepherd's Field on Christmas Eve!

I want to be filled with the awe and wonder that the Shepherds were filled with that night.

I want to have faith enough to follow a star out into the black night with full assurance that God will be there and take care of me on the way . . . to leave the "anxieties" of the world knowing that there is a more important realm of life.

I want to go to Manger Square!

In fleeting moments (far too few they are) I have known pure love, pure joy, pure happiness, pure fullness. Maybe there I will be enveloped completely in His love, His peace, His Spirit, His strength, that gives us strength to meet all that life brings.

I want to go to Bethlehem on Christmas Eve!

Dear God, fill us with Christlikeness. Only then will there be "on earth peace, good will toward men."

The time to leave the anxieties of the world and step out with faith into the "black night" lay ahead. Another year still remained to pray for the fullness of God.

11
Gaza: Part II

1971: Tensions

The Gaza strip in 1971 combined the features of a powder keg and a pressure cooker. It could explode at any time. With a population density nearing 1,000 inhabitants per square kilometer and a population growth of over 4 percent a year it fast became one of the most densely populated regions of the world. Of its nearly 360,000 Arabs, over 100,000 were Palestinian refugees crowded into eight camps. Hatred festered for the Israelis who displaced them from their homes in Jaffa, Lod, Ashkelon, Ashdod, and many uninhabited villages in 1948. They crowded into a "strip" of land only twenty-five miles long and four to five miles wide.[1]

The Egyptians controlled the Gaza Strip from 1948, and after 1967 the Israelis took over. Gazans found little consolation in the fact that many thousands traveled back and forth each day to work in Israel. A constant stream of anti-Israeli propaganda emanating from the Arab world encouraged the "shabaab" or young people to join the ranks of the "fedayin" or "al-Fatah" freedom fighters of the PLO. The older folks cautiously feared reprisals from the Israeli occupying forces.

To quell the PLO-inspired resistance, the Israeli Army called in its tough border police to Gaza. Its presence evoked fear, hostility, and passive respect. This special army unit was recruited from the Druze, Beduoin, and Oriental Jews. Each had their own historic grudge to settle against the Palestinians. Mavis watched as they made a "tough crackdown on the Fatah." They stopped people on the streets, searched them, sometimes pushed them around, and carried them away for interrogation. Later the occupation government began to move refugees out of the camps into new quarters. This step did not satisfy many Palestinian refugees who determined to return to their homes evacuated in 1948. They responded by declaring a protest strike of all businesses. The army countered by welding shut any shop that was not open.

The hospital staff felt the results of strikes and curfews. Staff members who lived off the compound could not make it to work on time and had to leave for home early before curfew started. The army detained some for questioning. Tension was the order of the day, but Mavis made scant mention of this in her letters home. She tried to encourage her family to visit the Holy Land in the spring and did not want to alarm them:[2]

Things are still rather quiet in Gaza since the occupying forces are taking a little tougher position with the terrorists and with the people. Our movements have not been restricted except when we might have wanted to move through a curfewed area. Then we are sent around like everyone else. Will it not be wonderful for the whole world if some of the troubled spots can find peace in the near future?

The Baptist Hospital compound had appeared as a haven of peace in the midst of troubled Gaza, but Mavis knew that compound living exerted its own special built-in tensions. The missionaries worked, played, prayed, and ate together. Frictions were unavoidable, especially with the political tensions outside. Being a single woman also added a special element. Singles need professional and emotional support as much as married couples. Mavis made a point of taking care of her own needs. She was careful not to make demands on the married men for what she could do herself. She enjoyed her independence. When a light bulb needed changing she did it herself. If the job was too big she called the maintenance crew. She filled her waking hours with work, entertaining the students, staff, and fellow missionaries, especially their children, enjoying her animals, and writing letters home. These activities offered her catharsis, as well as the time she spent in prayer.

The operating room was another matter for Mavis. There she demanded perfection, because she knew it meant a matter of life or death for the patient. Both students and doctors respected her thoroughness. When she said, "That's the way it is!" that's the way it was! She gained a reputation of canceling operations if there was no emergency, and the doctor made a habit of being late. The doctors began coming on time. Her real weakness, if she had one, was that she could not understand why the married staff did not have sixteen hours a day to spend in the operating room!

Family Visit

Anticipation of the "migration of the Pate family from Louisiana to the Holy Land" consumed most of Mavis's waking hours. Months ahead she wrote her folks about the weather, what to pack, and what to expect of the trip, encouraging each one to bring another person with them. "Now about packing and unpacking that suitcase," she instructed. "Yes, packing and unpacking, because you do not need nearly what you think you will need here. People are not so style-conscious. Wash-and-wear will do. So unpack two-thirds of your things so you can fill your suitcase with things for me, unload them here, and then fill that space with things you want to take home. Good idea, don't you think?"[3]

Mavis scheduled part of her vacation time to meet their tour bus and then bring them down to Gaza on their free day. She warned them ahead of time about shopping at the "tourist traps."[4]

Just let me give you a word of "for sure truth." When you go into a place with a tourist guide or with the bus driver you will pay more for what you want to buy than you do otherwise. The shopkeepers must pay the guide a percentage so they add this to the price. When and if possible you can usually spot what you want and then go back without the crowd and buy it yourself cheaper.

She tantalized them with mementos they could buy in Gaza such as hand embroidery, famous Nihad's paintings, and wool hand-woven rugs. She gave gentle hints of what she needed—eyelash refill, eye makeup, Sure-Gel, and film. But most of all she wanted to see them.

Finally the big day arrived, and she greeted Gwen, Genie, and Mattie with their group at the airport. They spent the next few days on a whirlwind tour of the country, visiting missionary and national friends and simply being together. Mavis toured them like a veteran tour guide and gave them perception of the people and customs. In Tel Aviv, she explained the Jewish kosher rules and why they did not get milk or butter with their meat. They spent the night on a kibbutz. Arriving late in Jerusalem for lunch one day, the Arab waiters were indignant. One muttered something in Arabic. Mavis responded in Arabic! From then on they waited on them graciously and even invited them home for a visit. In Gaza the janitor and OR technicians invited them home for a meal. They noted that the men did all the serving and clearing the table. Mavis told them, "When you get through eating, the family will have to eat what is left over!"

The days passed too quickly. After they left, Mavis reflected, "I think one of the biggest thrills of the whole visit was seeing Genie and Gwen together as sisters. I mean close together and to see both taking such good care of Mother. You do not know how much that warmed my heart."[5] The togetherness they shared was needed to sustain the separation to come. Mavis already longed for furlough in 1973. She thought of Aunt Mabel who missed the trip due to illness and sent instead "kicking-up-your-heels-money" for Mavis. The blue pants suit and white sweater they gave her made her the "jazziest 'misshy' in the Strip." How she missed the folks back home now that they were gone! She turned her mind to planning how she could meet Karen, her niece, who would be on a study tour in Rome in July.

One Saturday after Easter, following a marvelous Arabic feast at Dr. Sylvia Tarazi's home, two OR technicians came to Mavis's office. Mohammed and Ahmad had big wide grins on their faces. Mohammed said, "I think we have a recommendation for you."

"What?" Mavis asked.

Mohammed explained he had received two letters that week. "The recommendation is that your sister told to us to take care of you because she loves you very much!"[6] The local staff quickly became her family.

Technician Training

The OR technicians challenged and frustrated Mavis. Most who took her training came thinking they knew everything about the operating room. Her first task was to teach them that they didn't know much![7]

Mavis's reputation spread rapidly. The Dutch nurses at the Shifa Government Hospital invited her to train their OR technicians along with those of the Baptist Nursing School. She taught them strict compliance to sterile procedures. "Miss Pate," as the students called her, instituted a system of fines for infractions of the operating-room procedures. She kept a notice on the OR door requiring the wearing of a proper uniform on entering. A separate card for each doctor reminded the students of preferred techniques. One OR nurse humorously remembers the lessons he learned from her:

Miss Pate had a bell installed on the OR door. If you wanted to enter you must ring and wait until someone let you in. One day I forgot to ring. She said, "You are a good man; pay ten piastres! When you pay money you will not do it again!" One day I shouted. She said, "You are a good man—ten piastres!" I never shouted again. If you broke anything in the OR, you paid for it. She inspected for dust. One day she found a piece of cotton behind the door—ten piastres!

She enjoyed mixing a little fun with her work, and the students enjoyed it more. "We had a light schedule today so I gave some practical exams to my students on evaluation of technical skills, and then showed two films from biblical stories to the OR crew. They seemed to enjoy them. This afternoon at 3 the various technicians from OR, lab, and X-Ray played the nursing students in a basketball game. The Techs lost 28 to 24!"[9]

The hospital staff enjoyed the picnics most of all. Mavis planned a big affair for the OR crew, central supply and lab crew, and some special guests, and took them to the National Park in Ashkelon. This necessitated applying for permits for the bus and for all the people to travel into Israel. Many were refugees from Ashkelon in 1948, and this was their first time back. It went over so big that the OR crew decided they wanted to plan their own picnic for Mavis, just to show her they could do it.

Oh! The OR Picnic! This was one planned and executed by the 'boys.' It was Arab style. We had a half-loaf of Arabic bread with Kababs (ground and seasoned meat grilled on a skewer) inside. On the table cloth (which was leftover disposable linen from some disposable lithotomy packs) were whole tomatoes, cucumbers, olives, hot green peppers, white cheese, and labani. We were on a stretch of beach here in Gaza without a sign of shade and sand everywhere including in the sandwiches! There was "Gaza Cola" and watermelon.

(Being close to the students earned Mavis an invitation to an Arab wedding party. She noticed the difference from the ones in East Pakistan![11])

Went to my first Arab wedding. It was the wedding of the staff nurse who actually serves as assistant supervisor in the operating room. Actually it was not the real ceremony but a part of the festivities after the ceremony. During this portion the bride and groom sit in two chairs raised on a platform out where all can see them. Guests are all around them. Someone is playing the drum while they sing and dance around the couple. This honor is performed by the relatives of the bride and groom. The bride left the platform every thirty minutes and went inside to be dressed in another of her trousseau dresses and in her gold jewelry. Many friends are invited to return the following morning when the sheets from the bridal chamber are brought forth to prove the bride's virginity. Can you imagine? This is a real important matter in their family for community standing and reputation!

The arrival of Don and Patsy Meir during the summer lifted Mavis's spirits. Don was a medical student and Patsy an OR nurse. "We had two good days together in the operating room. What a joy that has been! I do not know when I have had the pleasure of meeting one of such 'like mind,' and it's great. I can take the trip to Rome and return knowing that things are in good hands." The Peaches's move back to Gaza following language study in Bethlehem also enlivened her. "Cari

Lynn and Jay liven up the place and Shirley is such a good 'coffee-mate' even if she does not drink coffee."[12]

August found Mavis in Rome where she linked up with Karen and a friend to tour the ancient city. Returning from the trip she found the operating room in good order and to her glee, Jo Anna Wright, the new journeyman nurse from Louisiana, had arrived to help.

Mavis looked forward to a long weekend in November when Ava Nell called and asked her to replace her as tour leader for six Arab female nurses. It was the end of the month of Ramadan, and they wanted to tour the holy places for the "Eid" or holiday. Mavis agreed only if the girls would help her write her weekly letter to her family. What resulted was sufficient reward, although not perfect grammar.

We are thankful for God that He gave us the chance to be together, and He gave us somebody to care for us while we are in our trip to Jerusalem. In fact we enjoyed our trip to Jerusalem very much. We had a lot of happy time as eating on floor as Arabic way, washing dishes together, cooking, and going to the cinema together. We enjoyed going to El Aqsa Mosque. Dome Rock, Solomon's Pools, Herodian's Mountain, etc. And how we enjoyed that trip very much, and we are very thankful for Miss Mavis Pate and Miss McWhorter and Miss Wright. We ask God to give us the chances to get knowing each other more and more.

Jacque

The OR technicians and friends were not all that spiced up Mavis's life in 1971. When Mavis climbed up the three flights of stairs to her "penthouse apartment" at the hospital she could always count on some unexpected surprise from Jacque. She acquired Jacque, pronounced "Jock," a little black dog of unknown pedigree from the Bivins family at Baptist Village. Therefore, Mavis said he was a Baptist, so he had to be OK! But Jacque tested her patience almost as much as the OR technicians. Fortunately Journeyman Don Roberts had a litter mate to Jacque and they were able to dog-sit for each other when Mavis had to leave Gaza.

Jacque held up, health wise, much better than her pair of pet parakeets. "Family speaking, I have three baby birds and an ornery dog. He loves to play rough house so he scares the little ones to death when he runs and growls." She watched patiently as the parakeets nested and the eggs hatched, only to see two sets of the baby parakeets die. Jacque stayed healthy, probably because he ate everything. Mavis remarked, "Have you ever heard of a dog eating cucumbers? Well, Jacque did, after leaving them lay for the first hour. He decided that was the only kind of food he would get so he ate them with a relish."

One had to be careful around him. Dr. Jean Dickman was having tea with Mavis one day. She had placed her plate of cake down to talk. When she got back to it, Jacque had eaten all but a few crumbs! He even liked the plants. "There is a constant feud between Jacque and the new plants in the house. He seems to think they should be implanted in the dirt the opposite way and insists on yanking them out of the pots periodically. Not so conducive to healthy plant growth."

Jacque was a very intelligent dog, or so Mavis thought. She had the carpenters install a new bookcase in her apartment. The only problem—Jacque could reach the bottom shelf. "It appears he has started to be a book worm. Surely, and he is eating them, and not reading them. He is just learning to talk, you know!" But Mavis's patience reached its limit when she forgot to feed Jacque one day. Upon returning to her apartment she discovered he chewed up one of her few pair of white nursing shoes! *Maybe the OR technicians are easier to handle,* she thought.

Financial Bind

A mounting crisis developed at the Gaza Baptist Hospital due to the changing financial situation under Israeli occupation. Workers from Gaza could make higher salaries in Israel and demand more pay to stay at the hospital. Others left for lucrative jobs in the Arab countries. Mavis described the desperate situation:[13]

We are having meeting after meeting trying to figure out how to work ourselves out of the financial bind that the changing economic situations of the work have led us into. We are going to have to cut down on the staff and find some other corners to cut. Maybe before it is over, we will have to cut down on the number of beds that we have in the hospital. Part of our problem is that our arrangement with the United Nations Relief and Work Agency does not give an adequate amount per patient bed that we can give care free of charge, and they are not in a position to increase it because the U.N. needs to divert much of its help to other more needy areas of the world, Pakistan for instance.

Mavis and the hospital staff chafed under a reality of institutional missions. "It is never difficult to get bigger, but to have to cut down is always a different story. VIPs from the Foreign Mission Board will be here the middle of next month to discuss things with us." The pressure of having to cut back caused natural strains in relationships with the hospital employees and between the missionaries responsible for the various ministries of the hospital. Baptists wanted to provide quality treatment. Quality costs money, and there was not enough money to go around. When quality had to be sacrificed it caused tensions between members of the mission team. Strategy meetings gave them the opportunity to plan in advance the steps to be taken, though Mavis complained that "the 'preacher bunch' show up late after I work all day and do double-time to get here!" Mavis had to pray a lot to face these problems. She shared her concern with family and friends in the form of a business meeting:[14]

Meeting was opened with prayer, my prayer that each of you are well and happy; that you are staying close to our Lord in thought and actions, that you are depending on Him for that which we cannot do alone, and knowing that He is all-sufficient to do that which you need. . . . maybe not all we want . . . but all we need. This knowledge I had to hold extra close to my heart today for the disappointments and loneliness.

Mavis was particularly disappointed when her assistant supervisor submitted his resignation to take a better-paying job in Bethlehem. Fortunately, he later reconsidered and stayed on to help her. Also, she got a "jewel" of a replacement for a nurse who was released. Through it all, she challenged her friends at the year's end, "Let's pray for each other more in the next year. I promise to pray more and to pray for all of you more."

Bangladesh

Throughout 1971 Mavis grabbed anxiously at every piece of news about East Pakistan (Bangladesh) and her friends there. Finally in April a letter arrived from Trueman Moore describing the situation after the outbreak of war. Mavis wrote her comments:

It was good to hear that Gloria is not having any trouble at all from her Hansen's Disease and is tolerating the medicine well. The whole family has moved to Orikandi, far out in the boondocks from Faridpur.

Trueman said the two Social Welfare Centers in Mirpur and Tongi were almost completely destroyed. The one in Mirpur seemed to be a target of wantonness and theft, the one in Tongi seemed to have gone with the surrounding houses. He said they were asked to leave Mirpur by armed men on two occasions. Conditions there are unbelievable, and it is questionable whether we will ever be able to do anything further. At this time none of our Christian friends have been killed, but many other Christians have in various parts of the country.

The Carl Ryther family updated Mavis on the situation when they passed through the Holy Land briefly in June. Her reaction to the news was "that situation should be impossible in a modern-day civilization but, oh how sad and inhumane and devastating and hopeless it is. Our's here is truly calm and mild beside that. We must pray constantly and diligently for Pakistan and friends there as well as the many other workshops of the devil in this world today."[15]

In October news arrived from Gloria Thurman. Mavis was relieved to hear that they had moved back to Faridpur and were engaged in church activities as usual. But this did not last, as the Bengali people fought for independence from the domination of West Pakistan. Full-fledged fighting for the establishment of Bangladesh erupted much to Mavis's alarm.[16]

I am so distressed for all our loved ones and friends in Pakistan. From all the news we are getting at the moment, it seems that they have not evacuated the internationals from Dacca. Rather in the news yesterday it was said that the plane to take them out was attacked and had to return to Bangkok. We must pray for our missionaries there, for our Christian friends, for all the multitudes in misery there, for the leaders that God may use them to bring about His will even though they do not know Him. Oh, I can only imagine the devastation this must bring to all in the path of the battles, and to all the country. No doubt, there is not enough food, or of any of the other necessities of life in the area. I pray for the Thurmans, McKinleys, the Bennetts, the Teels, that they be given strength and courage to meet whatever is required of them and in doing so, glorify the name of Christ and help others to know more about Him, even in these times of misery.

Her concern for friends in the new Bangladesh did not make her unaware of a great wave of danger that rose up around her. She kept closer touch to the situation than folks back home realized. She did not write them about her trips to the refugee camps at the invitation of her students. Sister Alice, Bible woman from the church, often accompanied Mavis on visits. As they talked and often prayed with the refugees, she felt their frustrations and heartaches. She asked Alice to teach her how to cook Arab food and to help her better understand the culture of the people she was fast coming to love.[17]

Deceptive Quiet

Amid renewed threats of war by President Sadat of Egypt, Mavis discerned a deceptive quiet creeping over Gaza, like the lull before the storm. Indicators were ominous. The local commander of the PLO was found dead in Mayor Rashad Al-Shawa's home, apparently from suicide. In November Dr. Merrill Moore asked Mavis to lay in six month's supply for the OR in case of war. Her newsletter, written in November, did not give any hint of apprehension:

It has been a good year in Gaza, one filled with good day-to-day work, hopes of continuing opportunity, challenges of obstacles and discouragements. I have tried to lead two departments in the hospital (Operating Room and Central Service) to a higher level of service, to guide nursing and operating-room technician students through a profitable and pleasant "learning happening," to tell about Christ in word and deed in hospital, church activities, and home, and to contribute to the planning and organizing of our overall work in Gaza. God has been the strength and guide.

There were encouraging signs at the hospital. Several Muslim students told her at the end of Ramadan, "This is not my Eid (holiday)," indicating to her their interest in the Gospel. They observed her quality of life and that of others in the hospital, and they respected it. Several Muslim friends put up Christmas trees as an open display of honor for Christ.

The fall season with Thanksgiving and Christmas around the corner reminded her of earlier days in Ringgold. Nostalgia set in. She pulled out the old record albums and dreamily absorbed their lyrics. Hymns by "Tennessee Ernie" Ford were a favorite. Even having her car stolen while on a visit to Bet Jala, near Bethlehem, and the cold wind and rainstorms of December spoiled nothing for her. Life as usual was filled with things of quality for her—cooking, people, celebrating Christmas. Mavis, despite her professionalism, had the golden gift of not taking herself too seriously. She kept a sense of humor. She laughed at herself when she went off to Tel Aviv to bring Dr. Andrew White back to Gaza for a concert. She forgot and left her cakes in the oven baking . . . overnight! It didn't spoil the joy she experienced at the baby shower for nurse Lenore Mullican or her delight when friends turned an "open house" into a surprise birthday party for her. It was December 23, 1971. She was 46. She exuded joy, despite a cold, drippy ceiling. Mavis spiced up life on the compound by wearing a new Dynel wig. She even invented, with the help of Mr. Abed, her cook, a new dish she called the "Nile Hilton Surprise," a spinach souffle, in which sauerkraut had mistakenly been added!

One event remained in the recesses of Mavis's mind, and she could not understand why. In the spring, the film *Bonnie and Clyde* was shown on the compound. Filmed in her native Louisiana, it told the true story that took place in her childhood. "I saw the name of Arcadia, Louisiana, on the screen, but did not see anything to make one proud. It was a ridiculous story, evidently largely fictional, and haunting in a way I cannot quite put my finger on. (What a flash this one was!)"[18] That haunting flash of the bullet-riddled car exploded into reality during the deceptive quiet of the New Year.

12

Gaza: Part III

1972: "Be Ye Therefore Perfect"

Saturday night on the top floor "penthouse" in quiet Gaza found Mavis exhausted. Her dog Jacque begged for another piece of hard candy from the Kerr fruit jar on the kitchen counter. He tried to attract Mavis's attention in order to satisfy his craving. She was worn-out. The Christmas and New Year's celebrations coincided with the Muslim and Christian feast days during the same month in 1971. An article for *Acteens,* the girl's missionary magazine, lay on the table waiting to be finished, but the aftermath of the flu sapped Mavis's energy. Thinking back over the past two weeks she realized that she overexerted herself.

Arabic style "high teas" and Bible studies for the OR and Central Supply crew required a cold drink, fruit, cake, and coffee. Then she served chili dinner for missionary friends. At least Mr. Abed cooked. *Maybe we ought to go in together with all our cooking since I have a cook. At least it would be cheaper that way,* she thought. The MKs were the most fun, especially at the Valentine banquet on New Year's Eve. The kids dressed in their Sunday best and tried to mind their manners for "Aunt Mavis."

Mavis's perfectionism and how she saw herself coming across to others concerned her. Mavis knew how much she demanded of people. Shirley Peach understood that Mavis was professional and a perfectionist. People who worked with Mavis had a mighty respect for her because she did everything so well. She knew what she was doing and how to do it. They never questioned her authority or professional abilities, but they did sometimes question her method of handling people!

As they were talking Mavis confessed, "I had to apologize again today. When am I ever going to learn?" she continued, "I want more than anything to be close to the Lord, but I am afraid to pray for it." Shirley assumed she prayed that prayer. She knew that Mavis wanted the ultimate experience with the Lord, similar to that recorded in the New Testament. They talked about the trauma that sometimes results in praying a prayer like that. Already the Lord had sent Mavis halfway around the world as a result of the prayer she prayed that day on the hillside in Glorieta, New Mexico.[1] In reflecting over this conversation, Mavis remembered the request she made to Bill Marshall when he counseled her about some minor problems. "Please pray for me," she asked, "I really desire a much closer walk with the Lord!"

Mavis sat, pondering these thoughts. Jacque playfully licked her hand, as if to beg for more candy. Mavis questioned, "I wonder what the Lord is trying to tell me?" She reflected on the series of chapel talks that Ava Nell had given on the 23rd Psalm. Somehow the words, "Yea, though I walk through the valley of the shadow of death, I will fear no evil; for thou art with me . . ." stood out in her mind. She told Ava Nell, "I really appreciated what you said. I have read it a thousand times, but that part of the 23rd Psalm has new meaning for me now."

Then, in typical fashion, Mavis's thoughts jumped ahead to the future. *Tom Nabors, the new hospital administrator, and Marilyn, his wife, will be here on the 20th. What am I going to fix for the reception? The McGlamerys and Anne Dwyer are leaving for furlough in Mississippi and Virginia. Maybe I can send some things to my folks with them. Come to think of it, my furlough comes up in the spring of 1973. What should I do? I think my best option is to study Arabic at the University of Texas. I sure cannot get any studying done here at the hospital! Gwen's idea of having an all-day open house with dinner on the table, is a terrific idea and will give me a chance to meet all my family and friends when I get home. Oh well, there's plenty of time to plan.*[2]

Jacque finally cuddled up on the couch next to her, his sweet tooth satiated. Mavis began to think about bed, too. *Should I work on that article? No, I don't think my mind is clear enough. If I don't feel any better than this tomorrow I don't believe I'll make it to church. Wish I didn't have to go to Tel Aviv to pick up that car! But at least it'll take care of my driving problem.*

The Lord's Day

The sky was gray, one of those overcast days that made Mavis ask herself if the rain would ever stop. She still didn't feel well. Ava Nell was concerned, so she went up to Mavis's apartment. She found Mavis typing letters to her family, making the typical carbon copies. "Why don't you let me go with Ed to pick up the car?" Ava Nell asked. She called Ed. He said it was necessary for Mavis to go because she must sign the papers. The car would be purchased in her name.

The white VW minibus was being prepared for the trip north. They removed the middle seat to make room for equipment that needed repairing and empty oxygen and nitrous oxide tanks to be refilled in Tel Aviv. It was getting late. Sundown came before 5:30 in the winter. Mavis mentioned to several people, "I wish I didn't have to go today. Oh, I really don't want to have to go today." As time came to leave she went back upstairs to get something she had left. On her way back down she turned as if she wanted to go upstairs again. Then she turned and walked out to the minibus. Sister Alice noticed that Mavis was wearing a hat. She thought, *Should I tell her to take it off on the way out of town, lest someone think she's Jewish?*[3] Arab women did not wear hats but usually dressed in a scarf.

Carol Beth, Mary Anne, and Joy Nicholas climbed into the back seat behind the oxygen tanks and arranged their bags and school-books. The trip to the MK dorm in Herzliyya took about two hours. Mavis settled into the front seat beside Ed Nicholas who was driving. Little Melissa Moore stood there with all the mission family and friends to give them the typical sendoff for the week. Mavis hugged Melissa and told her softly, "Remember, Melissa, whatever happens to me, I love you," and smiled.

As Ed pulled out of the hospital gate and sped down the street he realized it was dark and wished they were out of town. There had been an encounter that morning between the PLO and an army patrol near the Jebaliya refugee camp. Several PLO men had been killed. It was necessary to drive very near the camp. Mavis remarked, "Isn't it unbelievable how quiet it's been lately?"

The Black Night

They had barely cleared the outskirts of town when Ed caught sight of something out of the corner of his eye. Two shapes stepped out from the orange grove to his left. Suddenly, to his horror, he realized they were preparing to fire at the car! He shoved the accelerator to the floor! One volley of shots raked the vehicle at head level, the other at seat level. In a split second Mavis turned as if to shout at the girls to get down! She was hit in the head, chest, and thighs. She fell forward across the seat. Ed also was hit, but he tried to cradle Mavis's head in his arms and guide the car. With a tire shot out, he managed to maneuver the car several hundred yards down the road until it ground to a halt.

Carol Beth, the oldest of the Nicholas's daughters, grabbed the other two as soon as she heard the shots and pulled them to the floor. Bullets richocheted off the oxygen tanks, riddling the typewriter and schoolbooks around them. When the car stopped they saw that Mavis was critically wounded. With near-supernatural strength she tore a slip she found in her suitcase and wrapped Ed's leg and Mavis's head in a futile effort to stop the bleeding. Mary Anne jumped out and tried to wave down the cars going back into Gaza. No one would stop for her, perhaps because she was dressed in a coat with a tunic and they thought she was Jewish. Carol Beth walked down the road to the fruit-packing plant and tried to call for help. It seemed futile. She spoke English, Arabic, and French, but the Israeli telephone operator only understood Hebrew.

The group of Israeli soldiers on guard duty at an outpost several hundred yards down the road were especially alert because of the clash earlier in the day. Also, Ruth Dayan, wife of defense minister Moshe Dayan, was on a shopping tour in Gaza that afternoon and left only an hour-and-a-half earlier. Suddenly, they heard the staccato of the Kalatchnikov submachine guns and saw the tracer bullets streaking toward the car. Later, Dr. Merrill Moore described the details of the tragedy in a letter to Mavis's mother:[4]

The shooting was seen from a nearby army post and soldiers went toward the place and found the car and the people. Of course, those who did the shooting had run away in the meantime. The army called an army ambulance which came and took them all to the army aid station here in Gaza. From there the girls were able to call their mother at home. The army doctor saw the seriousness of the injuries and called an army helicopter to evacuate Mavis and Ed to the large 600-bed, excellently equipped and staffed Central Negev Hospital in Beersheba about 40 km. east of here.

As soon as the girls called Anne Nicholas, Anne called me. It was about 7 P.M. by this time. I checked with Dr. Roy McGlamery to see if he had any additional information, but he had not even heard of the attack. We contacted the army who came immediately. The deputy commander of Gaza came personally and took Roy and me in his car to the Army aid station where we saw the girls. They were in good shape so we sent them home while we made arrangements to go immediately to Beersheba. The helicopter had left before we reached the aid station, so we did not see Mavis or Ed. We took a hospital car and left for Beersheba. The officer sent his aide with us in our car to help in any way he could.

We arrived at the hospital in Beersheba about 8:30 and were informed that Mavis's condition was most critical, and she was being treated in the operating room by Dr. Tibeerin, chief of the neurosurgery department, and his associate. Both of these men are well qualified and had all equipment available to handle any problem within human power. Roy and I were not able to go into the operating room because of the intensive activity underway. The doctors were attempting to improve Mavis's condition enough that they could begin the actual operation. In spite of all they could do Mavis's condition became worse rapidly and, very soon after we arrived, one of the doctors came out to tell us she had died.

Ed was being X-rayed and we were able to be with him from this point on. The decision was made to operate on Ed but his condition was not serious. I placed a call to Dr. Hughey at the Foreign Mission Board in Richmond, but it was delayed in getting through about an hour. At that point Defense Minister Moshe Dayan arrived, having flown down from Tel Aviv in a helicopter with his staff. He came to find out about the situation and offer assistance. We told him we were having some difficulty getting the call through to Dr. Hughey. General Dayan took the phone himself and routed the call through military lines, so, very promptly I was speaking to Dr. Hughey. After that I was able to go into the operating room and be with Ed throughout the operation. In the meanwhile two of the nurses arrived, Ava Nell McWhorter and Bertha Jane Marshall. The military commander of the Gaza Strip, Colonel Enni, brought them over in his car. For at least two hours he was there with an aide. Also, the army chief of medical services of the entire Southern Command over the area from Ashkelon to the Suez Canal, with his deputy, arrived at the hospital about the time the helicopter came and remained with us until we left to return to Gaza at about 2:00 Monday. The chief of one of the surgical services and two of his associates operated on Ed. After the operation, Roy, Ava Nell, Bertha Jane, and I returned to Gaza to work on the necessary arrangements.

At every point we received the fullest cooperation from the military people and the hospital staff. To a man they expressed in a heartfelt way their shock, sorrow, and sympathy. Medically speaking, nothing more could have been done than was done. The best possible care was given under the best circumstances possible, by truly concerned doctors and personnel. I could think of nothing to do that was not done. The nature of the wound was such that there was no hope from the moment it occurred, yet everyone did all they could to ensure Mavis had every chance, every assistance, and everything which might even remotely benefit her. I sincerely believe she could not have been offered more in any medical center anywhere in the United States or anywhere in the world.

As soon as Carol Beth phoned her mother from the army clinic Anne Nicholas called the other missionaries. Those living out in town took their families to the hospital. They gathered the children and told them that there had been an accident, and Aunt Mavis and Uncle Ed had been shot. They huddled them into a hallway and turned most of the lights off. Not knowing the motive for the shooting they took no chances. During the night and into the morning they prayed and made plans for the funeral.

After receiving a call from Merrill Moore about Mavis's death, Dr. Hughey called Genie Norman in Minden, Louisiana. Mavis had left instructions with the Foreign Mission Board not to call her mother direct in case of an emergency. Dr. Hughey asked Genie to find out from the family if they wanted the body flown back to the states or to be buried in Gaza. He would call back in the morning. Genie called Gwen, and they both drove over to Ringgold to tell Mattie about Ma vis. Gwen knew that Mavis told her family when she went on the *Ship Hope*, "If anything happens to me, I want to be buried where I am." She made a point of telling every member of the family in front of her mother. Gwen's own philosophy, developed through many years of nursing experience, was, "I believe when you die, your spirit and soul leave, and your body is only a shell. I have seen people die with a smile on their face, and I know people who have had a premonition of death. Death is very hard for nurses to handle. For me to bring the body home was like bringing nothing but a shell." So they sat down with Mattie and agreed that Mavis should be buried in Gaza. They would put up a memorial monument in the Social Springs Baptist Church cemetery so that Mattie could see something tangible in Ma vis's memory. They conveyed this decision to Dr. Hughey, and he in turn informed the Gaza mission.

Back in Gaza the missionary family tried to sort out the details of the burial. "How are we going to get the body back across the border from Israel into Gaza? Where should Mavis be buried? The Baptist Church has no cemetery. The Protestant community cemetery has been desecrated by vandals, and we cannot imagine burying Mavis in such a place!" They finally settled on using a quiet spot behind the Nursing School. Merrill Moore described what happened:[5]

No one had ever been buried on the hospital compound. There is a law forbidding burial on private property. We approached the governor about his, and he issued a special order granting permission for Mavis to be buried here on the hospital compound. The entire mission met together to plan the service and other details, and it was our feeling that the most appropriate site for the grave was in a beautiful garden area behind the Nursing School. This is a quiet spot that can be kept well and beautiful. We felt it appropriate too that she be here near her work and her friends, both of which meant so much to her.

Still the problem of how to return the body from Beersheba to Gaza remained. They feared administrative red tape preventing this. The Lord took care of this detail, as Lenore Mullican discovered:[6]

Monday morning Ken took Anne Nicholas to see Ed in the hospital in Beersheba. Don, the journeyman, came in a microbus with the death certificate. He and Ken went to the morgue to complete papers for the permit to take the body. They showed them the body wrapped in a sheet and said they could take the body with them. So Ken and Don put her in the floor of the microbus. The middle seat had been removed. As they arrived at the Gaza border the border police checked Don's passport and waved them on. Upon arrival at the hospital they went into the mission meeting. The group was trying to figure out what they could do to get a special vehicle and permit necessary to transport a body across the border. They were shocked to find out Don and Ken had gotten past the patrol. Ken is convinced that God shut the eyes of the patrol so they did not know that they were carrying a body in the vehicle!

Mavis's death left Mr. Abed, her cook, extremely upset, but even as he wept, he continued to serve bitter Arab coffee to those who came to pay their respects in the sitting room of the Nursing School. He chose clothes which he knew were her favorites for the burial, a white blouse and a wrap-around batik shirt. They were easy to put on. Bertha Jane Marshall and Anne Dwyer bathed Mavis's body and dressed her. The simple, wooden handmade casket was covered with white satin. Her body was left in the chapel overnight. The Lord's day, in what Mavis called in a letter home, "The year of our Lord, or I hope it will be!" was over. She walked with Him through the black night.

Where the Bougainvillea Blooms

The weatherman predicted rain, but God graced Mavis's funeral with beautiful sunshine. The OR technicians insisted on being pall-bearers. As is customary in the Arab community they placed an enlarged picture of Mavis in a spray of flowers on the coffin. Dressed in white uniforms they bore her body into the chapel. The Arab officials and Israeli authorities who attended the funeral marveled at the calm and the joy they felt in the service. Ordinarily, such a funeral in the Arab community evokes weeping, wailing, and tearing of hair, and calls for revenge against the murderers! None was displayed as the resurrected Christ was honored by Mavis's sacrificial life and death. Dr. Merrill Moore eulogized her life in a letter to her family:[7]

Mavis's Christian witness was the motivating force of her life, and for this I appreciated her. Her witness was consistent. She did not have a Sunday Christianity and a weekday Christianity but always wanted to express in life and deed the high principles and commitment she felt. For Mavis, Christianity was not occasional great acts or pronouncements separated by periods of inaction and irrelevance. Expressing Christ's love as she knew it reached into every act and every relationship. After the funeral today someone commented that Mavis was always the same, going about her responsibilities in an orderly, methodical, reasonable way. This included her witness for her Lord, too. She did this in so many quiet ways that no one knows everything Mavis was doing in the Lord's name. As she went about her work she opened the hearts of her students and associates to the message of Christ. Several have expressed continuing interest and progressive understanding of the revelation in Christ due to the contact they had with Mavis.

Mavis was here because she loved people, but she loved people because she loved the Lord. It seems that she has died at the hands of those whom she was here to serve. Because Mavis was here in spite of the unpredictable, in spite of the dangers and ultimately became their victim, she will have a profound witness even in death. We pray that this witness will reach farther than Mavis ever dreamed of doing in life, and that the Christ who has given her eternal peace may give that peace to many others because of the life and death of Mavis Pate.

With eyes blinded by tears and hearts bound by grief, the OR technicians lifted the casket over their heads and bore it to the quiet spot behind the Nurses' Home. Only her "family" was at the burial site, the Gaza missionary families, and the Arab hospital staff among whom she served. Anne Dwyer saw the beauty despite the tragedy. "It was so-o-o warm and pretty at the burial spot after the cold church. I took special note. There is also a large poinsettia bush there and red geraniums around the inside of the fence. Some of the almond trees are also blooming." Mavis's family sent money for flowers for the funeral, but it arrived too late to take its place with the over twenty handmade wreaths and sprays given by local groups. Instead Ava Nell bought a bougainvillea vine and planted it near the grave. Its lovely red blossoms still shade the area, reminding others of the lifeblood that Mavis shed.

Many mourned Mavis in the United States. A wave of shock and disbelief swept the country among those who knew her. Memorial services were held at First Baptist Church, Tyler, Texas, and at her home church—Social Springs Baptist Church near Ringgold, Louisiana. Pat Haile drove all the way from Cayce, South Carolina, to meet Mavis's family and hear the Foreign Mission Board pay tribute to her on January 23, 1972:[8]

Dr. Cauthen and Dr. Hughey brought very meaningful messages. Dr. Hughey's Scripture was 1 Corinthians 15:50-58. He began by briefly reviewing the situation of the people of Gaza. Explaining how the refugees lived in poor conditions in the refugee camps since 1948, he said, "The present generation is born in Gaza with nothing to do but to sit and hate—for Gaza is a sea of hate in which the people live. But in this Sea of Hate is an Island of Love. Suddenly a great wave from the Sea of Hate lurched and took away a part of the Island of Love. Today, as evidence of that Island of Love, is a tombstone with the name Mavis Pate standing near the dormitory where I lived. Her grave will always be a testimony to the people of the Middle East, both Christian and Muslim.

Three hundred and forty-five persons signed the book of condolences at the funeral in Gaza. Among them were Victor Shimtov, Israeli minister of health, Abdul Aziz Al-Zuabi, deputy minister of health and friend to many of the missionaries, Brigadier General Izhak Pundak, military governor, many other military officers, directors of the nurses' association, dignitaries from Gaza and Bethlehem, and officials of the U.N.W.R.A.

This same kind of stone marks the grave in Gaza as stands in the cemetery at Social Springs Baptist Church.

MAVIS ORISCA PATE,

MISSIONARY NURSE,

DEC. 23, 1925 - RINGGOLD, LA. U.S.A.

JAN. 16, 1972 - GAZA,

"For me to live is Christ and to die is gain." Phil. 1:21

Dainty stars of allysium border the grassy plot in Gaza, giving a femininity to Mavis's grave. It is a memorial. She is not there. Mavis is with the Lord.

The Sea of Hate

The day after the funeral Ken Mullican found the badly shot minibus at the military government compound and drove it to Jarrell Peach's house. They washed out the blood, hair, and brain matter. To their horror, they counted at least fifteen bullet holes in the car! Then to their amazement Ken found a bullet lodged in the door on the driver's side in such a place, had it penetrated, it would have hit Ed in the head and killed him! Carol Beth saved the girl's lives when she pulled them to the floor. It was a miracle they were not all killed. They drove the bus to the hospital. Mavis's Bible was found, with the *Acteen* article she was working on tucked in it. What provoked such hatred? Was it revenge? If so, for what?

Indirectly, discreetly, the PLO sent an apology to the Hospital.

First to the funeral, then through the staff, a letter came to Merrill Moore, "It was a mistake. We have nothing against the hospital. We are very sorry. We were out to revenge the killing of two of our men that same morning. There was a curfew. We assumed that any car coming into Gaza was Arab, and any car leaving Gaza after dark was military or an Israeli civilian working in Gaza. Please tell your people not to drive after dark."

In the meantime, Shirley Peach inventoried all of Mavis's possessions. Mavis's meticulous lists of all she owned eased the process. Don Roberts took responsibility for Jacque. They grieved, for there was no replacing Mavis, as no human being can ever be replaced. Each is unique in this life and in eternity.

The staff immediately felt her absence in the operating room. Mission hospitals seldom have staff to spare, and Gaza was no exception. A couple of days after she was killed, Naomi, a nurse Mavis trained in the operating room, just came apart emotionally. She stayed away from work for two days out of grief. Ava Nell went to her and asked her, "Do you think Miss Pate would want you to be this way?"

She said, "No."

"Are you thinking of yourself or are you sad for Miss Pate?" asked Ave Nell.

"But, the OR will not be what it ought to be without her there," replied Naomi.

"Do you know where Miss Pate is now?" asked Ava Nell.

"She is with the Lord. One day I will see her!" affirmed Naomi. Under Mavis's witness Naomi became a believer. Mavis may not have known this before she died. The Island of Love was growing larger.

Two weeks after Mavis's death, Lenore Mullican, who just gave birth to her second child, took over supervision of the OR. She was amazed at how easy Mavis made it for her:[9]

I had very little experience in surgery and was relieved to see how well she had trained the nationals and how organized the department was. It was also obvious how very much everyone in surgery loved her, and it was an extremely difficult time for those who had worked closely with her. I felt it very important to keep things going the way she had done and especially to complete the training of OR scrub technicians which she had begun.

Ken Mullican, a laboratory technician occasionally slept in the guest room behind the hospital when he was on call. He thought it strange that the lab technicians seemed to discourage him from sleeping there. "Aren't you afraid to sleep up there by yourself?" they would ask. The guest room was behind the pharmacy near the carpenter shop. His curiosity at their caution was soon satisfied.

Early Easter Sunday morning in 1972, Israeli soldiers descended on the hospital compound. One mounted the stairs to the roof and shot off his weapon as warning. Then a mass search of the hospital took place. They summoned Dr. McGlamery to bring the keys. They came to a room they did not even realize existed, behind a row of lockers, near the place where Ken had been sleeping. The male nursing students also slept nearby. They pushed the lockers aside and found a padlocked door. "What is this room?" asked the soldier. Dr. McGlamery called for Ava Nell. She knew knowing about it. "I did not ever know there was a room here!" she answered. They forced the room open, revealing a basement room. A tremendous stench arose from it. They found the soiled bedding and a beautiful Quran. It was the hideout for two of the PLO cell group that killed Mavis! A nearby door led to the alley outside the hospital. Someone had been feeding them as they hid in the dark for over two months. Finally, the conscience of one of the boys hurt him so badly, because he was part of the group that killed Mavis, that he went out and turned himself in. He was not among the two that took part in the shooting. The army attempted to apprehend the others. One was killed and the other captured, tried by the military court, and imprisoned. The nursing students asked her missionary friends, "What are you going to do with the one that was caught?" One of the students said in typical Arab fashion, "You should go down and spit on him!"

Mavis's death shocked and disgusted the Gaza population. Their confidence in the PLO began to erode. Ken Mullican noted that there were numerous arrests, and it was over a year before another bomb exploded in Gaza. The attack on the hospital and Mavis so enraged the people that they began to overcome their fear of what would happen if they did not obey the PLO. Students in the past shied away from befriending each other for fear of being involved in the political struggle. Now a few began to share their faith in Christ with the missionaries, though they could not declare it publicly until they moved to other areas. The Island of Love kept growing.

The life and death of Mavis, as with untold millions of believers through the centuries, proved that *agape* love is immeasurably stronger than death.

13

Again: "Why Mavis?"

The Arab Christians express their faith in the resurrection of the dead by carving on their tombstones the saying, "He is alive and remains." They also refer to the deceased as "the one who has received mercy." Unfortunately, these religious cliches cannot answer the question, "Why Mavis?" Why was such a productive life snuffed out in its prime? Why the trauma to Ed Nicholas and his daughters, and to all those who loved Mavis? Why was she not protected? Was there a lack of prayer support back home? Each must find his own answer to these ultimate questions. God provides us with a few glimmers of truth, if we are honest with him. He is not afraid of our doubts, or our fears, or our anger over such a tragedy. He has been there before us.

A pragmatic approach to Mavis's death is expressed by Joseph B. Lewis, the son of Joe and Gwen Lewis, Mavis's sister. He was "Little Joe" to Aunt Mavis or "Ankle Bill," as loved ones in the family knew her. He penned these words as a memorial to Mavis but was unable to share them at the time of her death:[1]

This morning I have been struck by the amount of grief I have seen. I have heard words of sympathy for the bereaved, and in general, a feeling of sadness pervades the air. Now, I am not out to change the hearts and minds of men, but only to communicate a perhaps different idea from those I have heard so far. I loved Mavis Pate. She and I shared a rapport that went beyond words. She had a passion for living that swept up everything and everybody before her. She had a gift of laughter that completely destroyed all the petty little problems of the day. She believed that if you made fun of a problem it would either go away or get big enough to be dealt with. She walked with kings and humbled them. She walked with commoners and made them feel like kings. Her mark is set all over the globe, and where she trod, the land is beautiful. Flowers grow in her footprints. But most of all, she was an adventuress. There was always another hill to climb, another ocean to cross. In her the pioneer spirit was not dead. She saw in each new land, new challenges. Her soul was always alive to the world around her. She was, more than any other person I have ever known, a citizen of the universe . . .

Mavis Pate did not die young or before her time. She simply lived out her life faster than the rest of us! She did more and saw more in her life than the average person would believe possible. She died as she would have wanted to . . . dramatically, excitingly, and in a place of her own choosing. She did not die in a nursing home after a lingering illness, after a life of might-have-beens. She was where she was because she wanted to be there, and that is the whole story of her life and death. She did exactly as she pleased, and she did it with a happy heart . . .

And that brings me to my point. I rather suspect that she is up there watching now. If she is, she is bound to be disappointed that no one is smiling. She is pausing in her work of mending broken angels's wings to wonder what all the unhappiness is about. Let's face it. Who are we mourning? Certainly not Mavis Pate. She has achieved what every Christian desires. Earth is only a way-station, a mere rest stop between birth and eternal life. If anything, we should be joyous today. I realize that most people cannot. You see, the problem is that when we mourn Mavis Pate, we are only feeling sorry for ourselves. We are sad because we will not be able to enjoy her company anymore. She enriched our lives so we are all a little bit poorer now that she is gone. But look at the truth. She is not bothered with a tight girdle or a tight collar. She is not walking around with sore feet. She does not feel the cold or the heat. She does not have to put up with hard pews. She is not worried about inflation, pollution, crime, or whether she is late for an appointment. We are the poor suckers who have to put up with the little harassments of life, and *she* is the one who is comfortable. By being sorry she is gone, perhaps the truth is, we are sorry we are still here. Since I loved her so much, I can be happy for her, now that I have thought it through. I want to make a request. I want you all to smile. Smile at the joy that she has now attained. Banish thoughts of selfishness. Forget what you have lost and think of what she has gained!

Joe had no way of knowing when he wrote those words that God would literally fulfill them only a few months later. The life story of Mavis Pate did not end with the tragic attack on January 16, 1972. It only began.

The Unwritten Page

Some time after Mavis's death Dr. Merrill Moore reflected on the question, "Why Mavis?" He answered. "That is the unwritten page. There are things we just cannot understand now." Mavis's death caused great difficulty for the hospital staff. It was especially hard on Ava Nell. Not only did she lose her best friend, but she faced the crisis of how to staff the OR. She wrote a plea to her supporters in the states:

Oh, how I need your prayers. She was a co-worker who I could always depend upon for support and counsel. During these months I also learned to love her very much. I found her to be a true friend who I could talk with about matters of deep concern. I knew that I could always depend upon her to be a sympathetic listener who would never betray a confidence.

From a personal point of view this has been one of the most difficult things for me to accept that I have ever faced. I still cannot understand—why—; perhaps I never will during this part of life. Everyday I see new difficulties and vacancies left because of Mavis's death. The one thing that makes what still seems to me a useless tragedy possible to bear is the knowledge that God can and is using this for good. Indeed, everyday, I see evidences of the fact that her work and witness are not dead. I know that I for one am a better person because of her influence. I thank God that I had the opportunity to work with her, and after twenty years of being acquainted, to know her as a friend.

Ava Nell received notice from the Foreign Mission Board that Gaza would not be receiving any summer missionary nurses. It was a real blow! She replied, "I want to very honestly say that I do not believe there is any more danger here than any other place in the world today. We have every reason to believe that this isolated incident was definitely a tragic case of mistaken identity which is not apt to be repeated." She pled with the folks back home to pray for replacements. God rewarded her plea. Four summer nurses responded to the call, three of them graduate nurses![2]

An outpouring of generosity flowed from friends and churches in the states who wanted to give toward a memorial for Mavis. Over $8,000 came into the hospital for new equipment. The church renovated its building through donations. The little Social Springs Baptist Church gave about $200 to the Lottie Moon Christmas offering before Mavis's death. Now they give $2,000, and most of this from elderly members who are on Social Security. Northwestern School of Nursing in Louisiana established a scholarship fund in Mavis's memory.

The outpouring came not only in money but in lives. Tami Fields, MK, daughter of Bob and Eddie Fields, former directors of Baptist Village in Israel, was attending college in Georgetown, Kentucky, when the news announced Mavis's death. She spent the summer of 1974 as a volunteer in the Gaza Hospital. Beth Lytle, MK, daughter of Norman and Martha Lytle, current director of Baptist Village, served as a volunteer several times at the Gaza Hospital and later became a physician's assistant. Other young people spoke to their pastors about how Mavis's death influenced their decisions for the future. Don and Patsy Meir named their first daughter, born a year after Mavis's death, Laura Pate Meir.

A young Arab injured his hand in a work accident and came to the hospital for treatment. There Mavis and another nurse cared for him and shared the love of Christ with him. After Mavis's death he returned to the hospital and shared with Dr. Merrill Moore that he became a believer because of their witness. He later graduated from the hospital nursing school and became the head nurse of a cardiac unit in a major hospital in the United States.[3] Many new pages are being written!

"The Joy of the Lord"

Other new pages must be written. The burden to write the story of Mavis Pate remains because of the ongoing Palestinian-Israeli conflict and the sterling qualities of Mavis's life and her sacrifice. Mavis lived an extraordinary life and died a spectacular death. But there is much more. God gave a revelation of Mavis that impacted decisively on the lives of missionaries in Gaza and Israel. It was part of a mighty move of the Spirit of God that swept the Holy Land in the 1970s. What happened may enable us to understand a little more clearly, "Why Mavis?"

The Gaza Baptist Church invited Arab evangelist Dr. Bahjat Batarseh to lead revival meetings in September, 1972, after Mavis's death. Dr. Batarseh, a native of Jordan now residing in Lima, New York, played a key role in the renewals that took place in a number of churches in the area. When he arrived in Gaza, both local Arab believers and missionaries still grieved over Mavis's death. The personnel and financial crisis added to the tension at the hospital. Interpersonal relations approached the breaking point.

Dr. Batarseh felt the strained atmosphere as he preached. Few responded to his messages during the first few days of the meetings. Several of the missionaries told him, "We are in trouble with the Lord. We are nervous with the nationals and with each other." Finally he called for a special meeting with the missionaries.[4]

I shared with them the need for renewal and revival. The missionaries were losing their tempers and screaming at the nationals when they were not on time. They were losing their testimony. As I talked, one of the missionaries admitted that he was doing that. He began to weep. He looked at another missionary and said, "I hated you to the point that I prayed many times for God to remove you from this place. Will you forgive me?" The other said, "What is the point of my forgiving you. I will go and do the same tomorrow. You have to accept me as I am!" They both forgave each other. They began to weep and embraced each other. Dr. Lindsey's daughter had a special vision and renewal. She was shouting and dancing and praising the Lord. Dr. Lindsey said, "If God can do this to my daughter, he can do it to anyone!"

Pastor Ibrahim Hannah said the change in the missionaries was evident. "The thing that amazed me was that I sat back in the chair and did nothing. God did the work."

The impact of the renewal on Muslims convinced Dr. Batarseh that it was genuine. "Muslims began to come to the Lord. When I came back to Gaza later, Muslims were in the meetings. They asked for a private meeting with me. Each afternoon there were twenty-five Muslims who met to hear about the Lord," related Batarseh.

What really happened in that meeting with the missionaries in Gaza? What brought the renewal so suddenly after such a long period of difficulties? Shirley Peach shared the story from her perspective:[5]

None of us were particularly searching for the filling of the Holy Spirit until after Mavis died. It had been a hectic summer after her death. Bahjat came in September for meetings. He told us on Monday that he wanted to meet with the missionaries. Finally we met on Thursday night. Different ones had different reactions to the meeting. Some were "ho-huming" the meeting. I felt a bit angry. I thought he was going to get us together and tell us that women should not wear make-up or should wear far less jewelry. I expected that he was going to preach at us, but he did not. He started out by teaching us a couple of Scripture choruses. He quietly opened the Word and read a long passage about the Body of Christ and all of us being one in the Lord. He went on talking about it quietly and calmly. He told about how the Lord wants us to prefer one another and hold one another in higher regard than themselves. It was short and brief. Then he just stopped and did not say anything more. Everybody just sat there.

I was just about ready to leave, but I did not want to be the first. After what was to me a very long time, Ken Mullican spoke up. He said, very emotionally, "I am not leaving this place until I have a touch from the Lord!" He explained that every time he determined to get close to the Lord through Bible study and devotions, then something would come along and pull him away from the Lord. He just did not want any more of these ups and downs. So Bahjat said, "Do you want us to pray for you?" Ken said, "I want whatever it takes!" Bahjat began to pray and after several minutes of prayer, Lenore got up and just floated around the room, full of joy. She was having a vision of Mavis with Jesus. She saw that Mavis was so happy and beautiful. "I am ready to go now. I am ready to be with my Lord right now!" she exclaimed. Before she had been worried about her children and husband, but now she was happy, "Because I know now He is ready to take care of them in a way I could never take care of them."

One by one around the room almost everyone received an outpouring of the Holy Spirit. They were praising the Lord with inexpressible joy. There was reconciliation. Two missionaries that had been at odds with each other for years, and only a few days earlier had exchanged words, fell on each other's necks in tears asking for forgiveness. Others also forgave each other.

The next night we came together with a different attitude—with anticipation and joy. Those who had not been there the night before also experienced the touch of the Lord. We sang and praised the Lord.

The vision of Mavis broke the ice because we had all been feeling a heaviness because of her loss. We knew that she was with the Lord, but with the revelation, we knew she was happy. The test of the genuineness of this is that it had a long-lasting effect of reconciliation between the missionaries.

What part did Mavis play in the outpouring of the Holy Spirit that brought reconciling love to the Gaza mission? A key to understanding what happened that day in September 1972 lies with Lenore Mullican. What was the vision she saw? Lenore was unique in that she was an MK, the daughter of Dr. and Mrs. Robert L. Lindsey, veteran missionaries to Israel. Lenore grew up understanding Hebrew and Arabic from her childhood. She was quiet, petite, and pretty. After studying nursing she married Ken Mullican from Oklahoma. They came to Gaza to serve as a team, she in nursing, and he as a laboratory technician. She related her personal experience:[6]

In September 1972, Bahjat Batarseh came to Gaza and held a meeting at the Church on Sunday evening. I attended and knowing Arabic, I understood all that he said. He had been to our house and had asked me if I was Spirit-filled and I said, "I guess so," not really understanding what he meant. After my experience of being filled with the Holy

Spirit I realized that when you are, you have a definite "yes" answer. One year earlier Ken had stayed up all night praying and asking God for the power of the Spirit. He woke me up to pray with him and as I prayed the word "wait" kept coming to me. Later I felt that we were kept waiting in order to experience this as a mission group.

Also during that year Ken had seen a tremendous change in Ray Register and in his and Bob Lindsey's relationship and knew there really was something to the "Holy Spirit" experiences. He asked Ray to pray for him for this but felt nothing at the time.

As Lenore indicates, Mavis's death effected a dramatic change in the life of other missionaries, even in Israel. As a young, energetic, fledgling missionary, Ray Register chafed under the shadow of Bob Lindsey. He was the pioneer, visionary of the Baptist Convention (Mission) in Israel (BCI), and the acknowledged leader of the group. In addition, he was a noted Hebrew and Greek scholar. Register struggled to get B.C.I. permission to construct a church building in the northern Galilee village of Rama. Ray and Bob came into open conflict in mission meetings about this project and the philosophy of church development. The other BCI'ers tired of their outbreaks and appointed them as a committee of two to solve the problem outside the mission meetings. They jokingly called it the "Bob and Ray Show"! Some months after Mavis was killed, Bob and Ray set up an appointment to meet at Bob's little home at Poriyyah, above the Sea of Galilee, where he did his scholarly research. It was harvest time, and the wheat and barley covered the fields like a golden carpet.

As he drove down the winding road from Nazareth on the way to Cana, Ray came to the end of himself. Ray was tired of fighting. Ray told the Lord, "Lord, if I am wrong, help me to know how to change. If Bob is wrong, change him. Help us to agree!" Ray drove on past the village of Turan and came to the crossroad above Tiberias, then turned right toward Poriyyah. Just as he turned, the sight of the vast sea of golden grain on the sloping hillside overwhelmed him. He sensed something like a great sonic boom coming down from heaven. "Whump!" it hit the hillside. Then it came to him, "Unless a grain of wheat falls into the earth and dies, it remains alone; but if it dies, it bears much fruit!" These words of Jesus in John 12:24 reminded Ray of Mavis and her death. *How could my trails compare to the sacrifice that she made for the Lord?* he asked. He was ashamed of himself.

When Ray arrived at the little house in Poriyyah, Bob and he sat down and came to a solution of their problem within five minutes! Margaret Lindsey fixed supper and there around the table they broke bread and prayed. The Lord Jesus was there with us. He began a catharsis in Ray's life that went on for hours that brought him into a new understanding and love for himself, Bob, his family, and many others. The agreement they made that day became the basis for a church development program that was accepted both by the missionaries and nationals many years later. But the greatest thing was what it did for Bob and Ray's relationship. This was the change that Lenore had noticed. She continues her story:

Back to Batarseh; after the church meeting, he met in the small living room of the Moores with the missionaries. He told about the Holy Spirit and when he finished teaching us, Ken said, "I will not leave this place until I experience this which I so desperately need!" We had come through a very traumatic year and especially busy summer. Everyone was overworked and emotionally and spiritually drained. So Bahjat read to us some Scriptures. All the kids had fallen asleep in the other room watching T.V., even the babies, which was a miracle in itself!

As we prayed I felt like I was pouring out everything and talking 100 miles a minute. I raised my arms and could not put them down. Then I had a vision. I saw Mavis on the right hand of Jesus. I knew it was Jesus, but could not describe Him. My attention was on Mavis who could see what was happening in the room. She did not have to speak to me to know the reason for her joy was the experiences that were happening in that room. She impressed me as being *very happy.* Then I forced myself to look around me and come back down to earth, though I felt I could easily just go to be with Jesus. The scene I saw was the other missionaries hugging, crying, and asking forgiveness of each other for problems that had developed over the years of such close association.

I wanted to share the closeness I had with Jesus, so I knelt by each one and touched his hand. Ken also was filled with the Holy Spirit. With him it was a quiet experience but just as real. He would have liked an emotional experience, but God met him in a quiet way. I would have preferred a quiet experience, and God gave me a very emotional one, totally out of character.

The Lord confirmed the reason for Lenore's experience a year later:

One year later, I found out that Sarah Bivins at Baptist Village had a list written of prayer requests that Mavis had been praying for. At the head of the list was the request that the Gaza Mission be filled with the Holy Spirit! I then understood why God had allowed her to see us that day and why she was so happy. He allowed her to see her prayers answered.

Clothed in White

One final aspect remains to be understood as we ask with our human limitations, "Why Mavis?" It could include the ancient query, "Why do the righteous suffer?" Why Paul Rowden, Bill Wallace, Paul and Nancy Potter, Archie Dunaway, Roger Thompson, and Jim Philpot, to mention only a few from our own Southern Baptist past. These represent only a few of thousands from every church and tradition who laid down their lives for the name of Christ or who suffered undeserved and early deaths. It may be said that there have been more martyrs for Christ in this century than in any period since the first century. James and Marti Hefley in their award-winning book, *By Their Blood: Christian Martyrs of the 20th Century*, point out that the old concept of a martyr as one who is burned at the stake needs to be updated today:[7]

Martyrs of the 20th century have met their earthly end in more conventional, up-to-date methods such as gunshots, bombs, banditry, debilitating prison diseases, and starvation.

A second oversimplification is that Christian martyrs always die strictly for their testimony of Christ. This idea persists because accounts of martyrdom often do not include sufficient backgrounding of the events. When all details are known, it is apparent that most Christian martyrs die in circumstances *related* to their witness for Christ, for example . . . nurse Mavis Pate was killed by gunfire from a Palestinian refugee camp because Arab commandos mistook the Volkswagen microbus in which she was riding for an Israeli army vehicle.

So the dictionary definition of martyr—"One who submits to death rather than renounce his religion"—cannot always be strictly applied to the violent death of Christians. The second definition—"One who dies, suffers, or sacrifices everything for a principle, cause, etc."—is more inclusive. By this delineation Lottie Moon, the heroine of Southern Baptists, who died from self-imposed starvation in China, was as much a martyr as John and Betty Stam, who were brutally murdered by cold, calculating Communists.

If we take the New Testament and the teachings of Jesus seriously, each of us must be ready to suffer martyrdom if God calls for it. Sharon and Jim McPherson, Southern Baptist missionaries, placed themselves in the midst of a totally Muslim community in the Gaza strip. In a devotional talk before a Baptist mission group, Sharon pointed out that the question is, "Are you going to be a willing martyr or an unwilling one?" She quoted a statement that Jack Taylor made at the Elm Crest Baptist Church in Abilene, Texas, in 1983. "If God has marked you for martyrdom, all the angels in Heaven can't save you. If he hasn't, all the demons in hell cannot harm you!" Whatever the reasons for Mavis's death, God allowed it, and in the mysteries of eternity, He may have ordained it. Mavis was not only a perfectionist in the professional sense, as an operating-room nurse. She sought spiritual perfection in her pilgrimage with God. Her heart yearned for perfection, not out of pride, but out of a desire to be close to the Lord. Anne Dwyer, who knew Mavis well, said of her, "Mavis had been praying, seeking, and searching to know God better. He answered in a manner she did not dream of, ask, or realize. I am sure, like Enoch, she walked with God, and was not, for God took her."

The question "Why Mavis?" is also concerned with the meaning of suffering. Just as God in His divine wisdom allowed Jesus to suffer in agony and die, He also allowed Mavis to fall victim to the bullets of misguided men. Something redeeming resulted in both cases. In the first, Jesus brought through His death a new revelation of the resurrected life that liberates every true believer in Him. Mavis was in no way perfect like Jesus. She would cringe at the comparison. But her search for the reality of God, for the "bolt of lightning," for a perfection beyond reach, ended with the staccato of machine-gun fire. And something redeeming resulted. For the first time in years, Jews and Arabs laid down their arms and mourned an innocent victim who in many ways was too good to be killed. "What a waste!" some exclaimed. Maybe it was, humanly speaking. The redeeming story of Jesus' death still brings inspiration beyond understanding. Mavis, one of His imperfect followers, embodied the same passion, which challenges those of us who remain to count the cost. Reverend Bob Hamilton in a "Memorial to One of God's Children" put it so well:

God called a wonderful lady home! She is with Jesus today in Heaven. What a reward for a wonderful lady who loved and served Jesus with all her heart. There is no explanation for this terrible tragedy. God alone knows. However, one thing is clear. Tragedy steps into the lives of every person. No one is overlooked. We must be prepared when it comes. How can we be prepared? Simply by knowing Jesus as our personal Savior. To have Jesus in our hearts makes the difference. With Jesus in our hearts, nothing can separate us from His love; sickness, hatred, death, the grave. With Him eternal life and Heaven are before us. Mavis is in Heaven with the millions and millions of all ages who received Jesus Christ as their Savior while on this earth. What peace that brings to our hearts! Farewell, Mavis, we will meet you on that glorious day when Jesus returns! Amen! Come, Lord Jesus!
(Copied)

One last, fitting tribute to Mavis who gratefully wore the white uniform of a nurse and served her Master faithfully to the end is found in the Revelation to John on the Isle of Patmos:[8]

I saw under the altar the souls of those who had been slain for the word of God and for the witness they had borne . . . They were each given a white robe and told to rest a little longer, until the number of their fellow servants and their brethren should be complete, who were to be killed as they themselves had been.

After this I looked, and behold, a great multitude which no man could number, from every nation, from all tribes and peoples and tongues, standing before the throne and before the Lamb, clothed in white robes, with palm branches in their hands, and crying out with a loud voice, "Salvation belongs to our God who sits upon the throne and to the Lamb!" Who are these, clothed in white robes and whence have they come? . . . These are those who have come out of the great tribulation; they have washed their robes and made them white in the blood of the Lamb (6:9-11; 7:9-13).

Mavis inherited an honor bestowed on a growing number of those who die in the service of Christ.[9] God promised her a white robe. He will wipe away every tear from her eyes. Let us no longer weep, but let us gratefully enjoy His presence through His Spirit and willingly pay the price if He calls us to do so. The Lord will be pleased, and so will Mavis!

Postscript

After long and agonizing evaluation, the Southern Baptist Foreign Mission Board returned the Gaza Baptist Hospital to the Christian Missionary Society under the auspices of the Bishop of the Arab Episcopal Church in Jerusalem on January 1, 1982. It was renamed the "Ahli (Family) Hospital." Southern Baptists continue their medical ministry in Gaza through the operation of the Baptist School of Allied Health Sciences, which is located on the hospital grounds.

Mavis Pate is buried in the garden behind this building. Approximately sixty Arab young adults train in quality nursing each year at the school. Baptists continue congregational worship in the church on the hospital compound and minister to the wider community through the Library of Culture and Light in the city of Gaza.

About the Author

Dr. Ray G. Register, Jr., is a veteran of over twenty-five years service as a representative of the International Board of the Southern Baptist Convention in Israel. A native of Columbia, South Carolina, he grew up in Charlotte, North Carolina, and graduated from the University of Virginia.

While there, he received a call to missions and married the former Rose Mary Rich, a student nurse at the University. Serving as an officer in the U.S. Navy, he received the M.Div. degree at Southeastern Baptist Theological Seminary and pastored the Whitakers Baptist Church in eastern North Carolina.

Following appointment to overseas service in 1964, the Registers studied Arabic and Islamics at the Hartford Seminary Foundation, where Dr. Register later received the M.A. Degree in Islamics. After special studies at the Hebrew University of Jerusalem, he received the Doctor of Ministry degree from Southeastern Seminary. His doctoral project is published under the title, *Dialogue and Interfaith Witness with Muslims.* In Israel he serves as field evangelist in Galilee's Arab villages and specializes in witness to Muslims. He served formerly as chairman of the United Christian Council in Israel. The Registers live in Nazareth, Israel, and have three grown children.

Notes

Chapter 2

1. FMB Appl. (Foreign Mission Board Application), 5.
2. LH (Life History), 9.
3. Ibid.
4. FMB Appl., Ibid.
5. LH, 10.
6. Int. (Interview), L. V. Noles, 5/18/82.
7. Int., L. L. Wylie, 5/18/82.
8. Int., L. Sturbenz, 5/18/82.
9. LH, 11.
10. Ibid., 12.
11. Ibid., 11.
12. Ibid., 12
13. FMB Appl., 6.
14. Ltr. (Letter), C. E. Boyd, 6/3/67.
15. LH, 15.
16. Ibid., 16.
17. Ibid., 20.
18. Ibid., 21.
19. Ltr., W. M. Shamburger, 6/24/87.
20. LH, 22.
21. Int., Pam Lewis, 5/18/82.
22. LH, 23.
23. Ibid., 24.

Chapter 3

1. Mel Tari, *Like a Mighty Wind,* (Carol Stream, Ill.: Creation House).

Chapter 4

1. William G. Walsh, M.D., *A Ship Called Hope,* (New York: Scholastic Book Services, 1966).

2. Ltr., 8/85.
3. FMB Appl.
4. LH, 24.
5. Ibid.
6. Int., 6/17/82.
7. Ltr., 3/20/63.
8. FMB Appl., 2.
9. Ibid., 4.
10. Ibid., 6.
11. FMB Appl., 2/28/64, 5/4/64.
12. FMB Appl.
13. Ltr., 1/11/65.

Chapter 5

1. Ltr., 2/5/65.
2. Ibid., 2/7/65.
3. D. (Diary), 9/5/65.
4. Ibid., 3/5/65.
5. Ltr., 2/24/65.
6. D., 3/14/65.
7. Ltr., 3/14/65.
8. Ibid., 4/2/65.
9. D. 3/31/65.
10. Ibid., 3/22/66.
11. Newsletter, 6/1/65.
12. D. 4/13/65.
13. Ltr., G. P. Thurman, 12/3/82.
14. D., 5/17/65.
15. Ltr., 8/7/65.
16. Thurman, Ibid.
17. Ltr., 5/30/65.
18. D., 10/31/65.
19. Ibid., 11/16/65.
20. Ibid., 12/19/65.
21. Ltr., 3/21/65.

22. Ibid., 2/18/66.
23. D., 1/24/66.
24. Ltr., 3/26/66.
25. Ibid., 5/22/66.
26. Ibid., 6/12/66.
27. Ibid., 7/10/66.
28. Ibid., 7/3/66.
29. Ibid., 7/28/66.
30. Ibid., 8/28/66.
31. Ibid., 8/28/66.
32. Ibid., 9/25/66.
33. Ibid., 10/1/66.
34. D., 11/2/66.

Chapter 6
1. Ltr., 10/10/66.
2. Ibid.
3. D., 11/2-3/66.
4. Ibid., 11/15/66.
5. Ltr., 11/13/66.
6. Ibid., 11/27/66.
7. Ibid., 12/6/66.
8. Ibid., 12/17/66.
9. Ibid., 12/66.
10. Keith Miller, *The Taste of New Wine* (Waco, Tex.: Word, Inc., 1965).
11. Ltr., 12/6/66
12. D., 1/12/67.
13. Ltr., 1/26/67.
14. Ibid., 2/4/67
15. *National Geographic*, Vol. 131, No. 1, January, 1967, 9,26.
16. G. P. Thurman, 12/3/82.
17. Ltr. 2/25/67.
18. Ibid., 12/3/82.
19. Ibid., 3/4/67.
20. Ibid., 3/22/67.
21. Ibid.
22. Ibid.
23. D., 1/15/67.
24. Ibid., 3/21/67.

Chapter 7
1. D., 3/27—4/11/67.
2. Ltr., G. Thurman, 3/12/82.
3. Ltr., 5/14/67.
4. Ibid.
5. Ibid.
6. Ibid., 6/12/67.
7. Ltr., 7/14/67.
8. Ltr., 9/17/67.
9. Ibid., 1/14/68.
10. Ibid., 2/7/68.
11. John 6:35.
12. Ltr., P. Haile, 1982.
13. Ibid.
14. Ibid.

Chapter 8
1. Ltr., G. Norman, 8/22/86.
2. *Encyclopedia Britannica*, 1973, Vol. 13, Vol. 14, *356.*
3. *Southern Baptist Convention Annual, 1968,* 76.
4. Int., Z. Meachum, 5/8/82.
5. G. Norman, Ibid.

Chapter 9
1. Ltr., 3/19/69.
2. Ibid., 3/28/69.
3. Ibid., 4/4/69.
4. Ibid., 4/14/69.
5. Ibid.
6. Ibid., 7/11/69.
7. Ibid., 9/21/69.
8. Ibid., 10/19/69.
9. Ltr., J. McKinley, 3/16/86.
10. Ibid.
11. Ltr., 1/11/70.
12. Ltr., 1/31/70.

Chapter 10
1. Int., A. N. McWhorter, 9/5/82.
2. Int., J. Yates, 8/16/85.
3. Ltr., 2/24/70.
4. Ibid., 3/11/70.
5. Ibid., 4/24/70.
6. Ibid., 6/14/70.

7. Ibid., 7/6/70.
8. Ibid., 7/12/70.
9. McWhorter, Ibid.
10. Ltr., 8/30/70.
11. Ibid., 9/13/70.
12. Ibid., 10/11/70.
13. Ibid., 10/18/70.
14. Ibid., 10/22/70.
15. Ibid., 12/6/70.
16. Watchman Nee, *The Release of the Spirit* (Sure Foundation, 1965).
17. Ltr., 12/20/70.

Chapter 11
1. Avraham Katz-Oz, "Why the problem of Gaza is separate," *Jerusalem Post,* Sun. Aug. 17, 1986, 8.
2. Ltr., 1/24/71.
3. Ibid., 1/11/71.
4. Ibid., 1/30/71.
5. Ibid., 3/26/71.
6. Ibid., 4/11/71.
7. Ibid., 2/21/71.
8. Int., M. Ali, 9/1/87.
9. Ltr., 2/25/71.
10. Ibid., 7/4/71.
11. Ibid., 9/13/70.
12. Ibid., 7/11/71.
13. Ibid., 10/3/71.
14. Ibid., 10/31/71.
15. Ibid., 6/20/71.
16. Ibid., 12/7/71.
17. Ltr., A. N. Anton, 11/26/87.

Chapter 12
1. Int., Shirley Peach, 8/25/82.
2. Ltr., 1/15/72.
3. Anton, Ibid.
4. Ltr., Dr. Merrill Moore, 1/18/72.
5. Ibid.
6. Ltr., Lenore Mullican, 12/24/84.
7. Ltr., 1/18/72.
8. Ltr., Pat Haile, 1982.
9. Mullican, Ibid.

Chapter 13
1. Lt., Joseph B. Lewis, 1/23/72.
2. Ltr., A. N. McWhorter, 2/14/72.
3. James and Marti Hefley, *By Their Blood: Christian Martyrs of the 20th Century* (Mott Media, 1979), 334.
4. Int., Bahjat Batarseh, 8/8/86.
5. Shirley Peach, Ibid.
6. Mullican, Ibid.
7. Hefley, Ibid., vii-viii.
8. Rev. 6:9,11; 7:9,14 (RSV)
9. Ltr., John Bray, 2/26/88.